ISOMETRIC EXERCISE FOR HIGH BLOOD PRESSURE

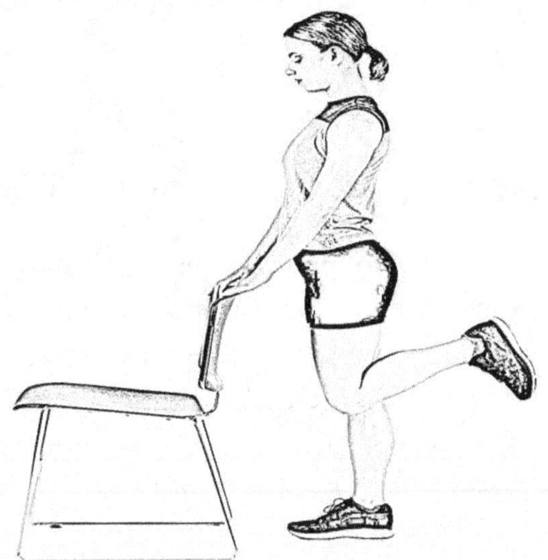

Enhancing Cardiovascular Health Through Static Exercises

Weaver Vancamp

TABLE OF CONTENTS

Introduction 7

CHAPTER 1 9

Knowing More About Isometric Exercise 9

What Is Isometric Exercise? 9

The Science Behind Isometric Exercise 12

How Isometric Exercise Differs from Other Types of
Exercise? 18

Benefits of Isometric Exercise 24

CHAPTER 2 31

Understanding High Blood Pressure 31

What Is High Blood Pressure (Hypertension) 31

Causes and Risk Factors of Hypertension 33

The Dangers of Untreated Hypertension to Health ... 39

CHAPTER 3 46

The Connection Between Isometric Exercise and Blood
Pressure 46

How Isometric Exercise Helps Lower Blood Pressure ... 46

The Role of Muscle Contraction in Cardiovascular Health
.... 53

Research and Studies Supporting Isometric Exercise for
Hypertension 58

CHAPTER 4 65

Getting Started with Isometric Exercise 65

Who Should Perform Isometric Exercises 65

Safety Guidelines and Precautions 71

Recommended Equipment for Isometric Training.............75

Frequency and Duration of Workouts..............................81

CHAPTER 5 84

Types of Isometric Exercises for High Blood Pressure 84

Upper Body Exercises..84

Wall push-ups 84

Doorway push-ups 87

Plank 90

Isometric bicep curls 92

Isometric triceps extensions 94

Isometric shoulder press..98

Isometric lat pulldowns..101

Isometric chest press 104

Isometric overhead press......................................108

Isometric row 112

Lower Body Exercises 116

Wall sit...116

Calf raises...119

Hamstring curls..122

Glute bridge 125

Isometric leg extensions.......................................128

Isometric leg curls..131

Isometric quadriceps contractions.......................134

Isometric inner thigh contractions.......................137

Isometric outer thigh contractions.......................140

Isometric hip abductions 143

Core Exercises 146

Boat pose... 146

Side plank.. 149

Isometric plank...................................... 152

Isometric bicycle crunches.................... 155

Isometric leg raises 158

Isometric Russian twists........................ 161

Isometric hip thrusts.............................. 164

Isometric pelvic tilts.............................. 167

Isometric oblique twists 170

Isometric bridge holds........................... 173

CHAPTER 6 176

Creating a Isometric Exercise Routine............................. 176

Progressing Your Workouts Safely............................. 176

Combining Isometric Exercise with Other Forms of
Physical Activity 178

CHAPTER 7 181

Monitoring Blood Pressure While Exercising 181

How to Measure Blood Pressure Accurately 181

Tracking Your Progress with Isometric Exercise 183

Recognizing Signs of Improvement............................ 185

CHAPTER 8 187

Lifestyle Modifications to Support Lower Blood Pressure
.... 187

The Role of Diet in Hypertension Management 187

Stress Management and Its Impact on Blood Pressure 189

Sleep and Rest for Cardiovascular Health 191

CHAPTER 9 193

Special Considerations for Specific Populations 193

Isometric Exercise for Seniors 193

Isometric Exercise for Those with Heart Conditions ... 195

Modifications for Individuals with Limited Mobility .. 197

CHAPTER 10 199

Frequently Asked Questions (FAQ) 199

Common Misconceptions About Isometric Exercise ... 199

Can Isometric Exercise Replace Medication for
Hypertension? 201

How Long Until You See Results? 203

CHAPTER 11 205

Conclusion 205

Introduction

Are you someone with high blood pressure who's been advised to incorporate exercise into your daily routine but don't know where to start? If so, you're not alone. High blood pressure, also known as hypertension, is a widespread health concern that affects millions of people globally. It is a silent condition, often with no obvious symptoms, but its impact on heart health can be life-threatening if left unmanaged. While medication and dietary changes are essential, exercise remains one of the most powerful, natural tools for controlling hypertension. But with so many types of exercises out there, which one is right for you, especially if you're concerned about overexerting yourself?

Enter **isometric exercises**—a lesser-known, but highly effective form of exercise that could be the solution you're looking for. Isometric exercises involve holding your muscles in a static contraction without moving the surrounding joints. These exercises are not as physically intense as traditional dynamic exercises like running or lifting weights, but they can still provide significant cardiovascular benefits. Studies have shown that regular isometric training can help reduce blood pressure, improve muscle strength, and enhance overall cardiovascular health, making it a great choice for people with hypertension.

What makes isometric exercises particularly beneficial for those with high blood pressure is that they allow you to engage muscles without overstressing your heart or straining your joints. Unlike aerobic exercises, which can cause spikes in heart rate and blood pressure during high-intensity activity, isometric exercises keep your body stable while your muscles do the work, promoting steady circulation and reducing stress on your cardiovascular system. Plus, these exercises are low-impact, easy to perform anywhere, and don't require any special equipment, making them accessible to almost everyone, regardless of fitness level.

In this book, we will dive deeper into the science behind how isometric exercises can specifically help lower blood pressure. You'll learn about various exercises that target different muscle groups, how to safely incorporate them into your daily routine, and why consistency is key to seeing real results. Whether you're just starting your fitness journey or looking for a safer way to exercise with hypertension, this guide will give you the tools and confidence you need to improve your health through the power of isometric exercise.

CHAPTER 1

Knowing More About Isometric Exercise

What Is Isometric Exercise?

Isometric exercise is a type of strength training in which the muscles are engaged without movement. Unlike traditional exercises, where you lift, push, or pull weights through a range of motion, isometric exercises involve holding a static position. The term "isometric" comes from the Greek words "iso," meaning equal, and "metric," meaning measure—referring to the fact that the length of the muscle doesn't change during the exercise. While there is no visible movement in the body, the muscles are working hard to maintain a contracted state, generating tension and building strength.

How Does Isometric Exercise Work?

In isometric exercises, your muscles contract to hold a position rather than move a load. Imagine holding a plank, a wall sit, or pressing your palms together in front of your chest. In each of these cases, your muscles are fully engaged, but your joints aren't moving. The key is muscle contraction—when you tighten your muscles and hold them in a fixed position for a certain amount of time.

There are two types of muscle contractions that occur during exercise: concentric and eccentric. Concentric contraction happens when a muscle shortens as it exerts force (e.g., lifting a dumbbell during a biceps curl).

Eccentric contraction happens when a muscle lengthens under tension (e.g., lowering the dumbbell back down). Isometric contractions, however, fall into a unique category. They generate force without changing the muscle length or causing visible movement. This makes isometric exercises ideal for situations where stability and endurance are more important than dynamic movement, such as holding a position during a wall sit or keeping your body in a plank position.

Examples of Isometric Exercises

Isometric exercises come in many forms and can be performed with or without equipment. Common examples include:

- **Plank:** Holding your body in a straight line, supported by your forearms and toes.
- **Wall Sit:** Sitting against a wall with your legs bent at a 90-degree angle, as though sitting in a chair.
- **Handgrip Squeeze:** Squeezing a grip trainer or even just your hands together to engage the muscles of your forearms and hands.
- **Isometric Squat Hold:** Squatting down and holding the position without moving up or down.

Even though these exercises may appear simple, they can be incredibly challenging as they require prolonged muscle engagement, which builds endurance and strength over time.

Why Choose Isometric Exercise?

If you're looking for a form of exercise that is low-impact yet highly effective, isometric training might be the perfect choice. It's especially suitable for individuals who may not be able to engage in high-intensity workouts or who need a safe and manageable way to strengthen their muscles. Since these exercises can be easily modified, they are accessible to people at all fitness levels.

Another reason isometric exercises are gaining attention is due to their ability to target specific muscle groups without putting excess strain on the heart and joints. For people managing conditions like high blood pressure, this balance between strength and safety is critical. Isometric exercises allow you to challenge your muscles while maintaining control over your breathing and heart rate, preventing spikes that could be harmful for individuals with cardiovascular concerns.

Isometric Exercise and Mental Focus

An often-overlooked benefit of isometric exercises is the mental focus they require. Holding a position for a prolonged period demands concentration, mindfulness, and control over your breathing. As a result, isometric training can also serve as a form of mental conditioning. By focusing on holding the position and controlling muscle tension, many people find that they build greater mental discipline, which can transfer into other areas of life, including stress management—another important factor in blood pressure control.

Isometric exercise is a unique and scientifically backed form of physical activity that engages muscles without causing movement in the joints. While this type of exercise might seem less dynamic than traditional workouts like running, lifting, or cycling, its effectiveness lies in how it impacts muscle fibers, nervous system engagement, and even cardiovascular health. To fully appreciate how isometric exercises work, it's important to understand the physiological mechanisms behind them and how these exercises can contribute to strength development, endurance, and even blood pressure regulation.

What Happens During an Isometric Contraction?

When you perform an isometric exercise, your muscles generate force without changing length. This is different from the two types of contractions you might be more familiar with—**concentric** (where the muscle shortens) and **eccentric** (where the muscle lengthens). In an isometric contraction, the muscle is activated, but it doesn't move. Think of holding a weight in a fixed position or maintaining a plank for an extended period: your muscles are engaged, but there's no visible movement.

During isometric exercises, your muscles contract by activating motor units within muscle fibers. Motor units consist of a motor neuron and the skeletal muscle fibers it controls. When a motor neuron sends a signal, it triggers the muscle fibers to contract. In an isometric contraction, multiple motor units are engaged to maintain muscle tension, and the muscle fibers are continually working to hold the position. The longer you maintain the position, the more muscle fibers become involved, which builds muscle endurance over time.

Neuromuscular Adaptations

One of the key components of isometric exercise is how it enhances **neuromuscular efficiency**. Neuromuscular efficiency refers to the ability of the nervous system to effectively communicate with muscles to produce the desired force. In isometric training, this communication improves as you hold a position for an extended time. The brain sends continuous signals to the muscles to maintain tension, which strengthens the neuromuscular connections over time. This process helps increase both muscular strength and endurance.

The static nature of isometric exercises allows for focused recruitment of specific muscle fibers, particularly the type I muscle fibers (slow-twitch), which are used for endurance. These fibers are more resistant to fatigue, making them essential for prolonged muscle contractions. By repeatedly engaging these fibers in static holds, you improve your muscle's ability to sustain contractions without fatiguing, which can be particularly beneficial for improving posture, stability, and functional strength.

Muscle Fiber Activation and Strength Development

While isometric exercises don't involve the same range of motion as dynamic exercises, they can still lead to significant gains in muscle strength. This is due to the high degree of **muscle fiber recruitment** that occurs during isometric contractions. When you hold a position, your muscles are forced to recruit more motor units to maintain the tension over time. The greater the tension, the more motor units are activated, which leads to strength improvements.

Research has shown that **isometric exercises** can increase strength in specific joint angles where the contraction occurs. For example, holding a squat position will strengthen the muscles at the angle you hold. Over time, this can lead to increased strength in those muscles, even though there's no movement involved during the exercise.

How Isometric Exercises Impact Blood Pressure

One of the most significant benefits of isometric exercises, particularly for individuals with high blood pressure, is their effect on cardiovascular health. Numerous studies have indicated that isometric training can lead to reductions in both **systolic** and **diastolic** blood pressure. This is particularly valuable for individuals who may not be able to engage in high-intensity aerobic exercises, which can sometimes elevate blood pressure during the activity.

The **mechanism** behind the blood pressure-lowering effect of isometric exercise is still being studied, but there are several hypotheses:

1. **Increased Vascular Health:** Isometric exercises can enhance vascular function by improving

endothelial health. The endothelium is the inner lining of blood vessels, and when it functions properly, it helps regulate blood pressure by allowing blood vessels to dilate and constrict as needed. By improving endothelial function, isometric exercises may contribute to better blood flow and lower blood pressure.

2. **Reduced Sympathetic Nervous System Activity:** The sympathetic nervous system is responsible for the "fight or flight" response, which can elevate heart rate and blood pressure. Regular isometric training may reduce sympathetic activity over time, leading to lower resting blood pressure. This adaptation is particularly beneficial for individuals with hypertension, as it allows the cardiovascular system to operate more efficiently at rest.

3. **Improved Autonomic Control:** Isometric exercises may also improve the balance between the **sympathetic** (fight or flight) and **parasympathetic** (rest and digest) branches of the autonomic nervous system. By enhancing parasympathetic activity, isometric exercises can help lower resting heart rate and blood pressure, contributing to better cardiovascular health overall.

Muscle Tension and Metabolic Demand

During isometric exercise, the sustained muscle contraction creates a steady demand for energy. Even though the body isn't moving, the muscles require ATP (adenosine triphosphate) to maintain the contraction. This increased **metabolic demand** can improve muscle endurance and overall metabolic health, making isometric exercises an effective way to boost both strength and energy use without the high intensity of traditional aerobic workouts.

Because the muscles are continuously contracted, isometric exercises can also lead to an increase in **muscle tone** over time. When done consistently, they enhance muscle definition without the need for heavy weights or high-impact activities.

Oxygen Consumption and Breathing Techniques

Although isometric exercises are less dynamic than other forms of exercise, they still impact **oxygen consumption**. Holding a contraction requires your muscles to utilize oxygen to sustain energy production. Learning proper **breathing techniques** during isometric exercise is crucial for maximizing results and reducing strain on the cardiovascular system.

Many beginners tend to hold their breath while performing isometric exercises, a phenomenon known as the **Valsalva maneuver**. However, holding your breath can cause spikes in blood pressure, which is counterproductive for individuals trying to manage hypertension. Instead, focusing on steady, controlled breathing during isometric holds ensures that oxygen is continuously delivered to the muscles, allowing for sustained contractions and a more relaxed cardiovascular response.

By incorporating **controlled breathing** into your isometric routine, you can reduce stress on your heart and make the exercise safer and more effective, particularly for those managing high blood pressure.

When it comes to exercise, there are many forms to choose from—whether you're looking to build strength, improve cardiovascular health, or enhance flexibility. Among the various options, **isometric exercise** stands out for its unique approach to muscle engagement. Unlike traditional forms of exercise, where your muscles go through a range of motion, isometric exercises involve holding a static position, engaging the muscles without movement. But how exactly does this type of exercise differ from others, and what makes it particularly beneficial for certain fitness goals, like managing high blood pressure? Let's explore.

1. Static vs. Dynamic Movements

The most significant difference between isometric exercise and other types of exercise lies in the way muscles are worked.

- **Isometric Exercise:** In isometric exercises, the muscle contracts but does not change length, and there is no visible movement in the joints. The focus is on maintaining tension in a static position for a certain duration. For example, holding a plank or sitting against a wall in a squat position are common isometric exercises. The goal is to keep the muscle contracted for as long as possible, which builds endurance and strength in a very controlled manner.

- **Other Types of Exercise:** In contrast, traditional strength exercises—like weight lifting, running, or cycling—are dynamic. These exercises involve **concentric** contractions (muscles shortening as they lift or push) and **eccentric** contractions (muscles lengthening as they lower or release). Dynamic movements improve muscle strength, flexibility, and cardiovascular fitness through repeated motions that stretch and contract the muscles in varying ranges of motion.

The key takeaway here is that isometric exercises offer a more controlled form of muscle engagement without the wear and tear of repetitive movements, making them ideal for individuals with joint issues or those managing high blood pressure.

2. Intensity and Impact on Joints

Another area where isometric exercise differs is in its impact on the joints and overall intensity.

- **Low Impact Nature of Isometric Exercise:** Since isometric exercises do not involve joint movement, they are much gentler on your joints compared to other exercises that require bending, twisting, or impact. For this reason, isometric exercises are a popular choice for people with arthritis, joint pain, or those recovering from injuries. Holding positions like a plank or wall sit places tension on the muscles without causing repetitive strain to the knees, hips, or back.

- **Other Types of Exercise:** Dynamic exercises, such as running or weightlifting, often place significant stress on joints because of the repetitive movement involved. While these exercises are fantastic for building muscle and improving cardiovascular health, they may not be suitable for everyone, especially those with joint issues or those recovering from surgeries or injuries.

This reduced strain on the joints makes isometric exercises a safe alternative for people who might otherwise avoid exercise due to pain or mobility issues.

3. Cardiovascular Impact and Blood Pressure

One of the key reasons people look to isometric exercises, especially for managing high blood pressure, is their distinct cardiovascular impact.

- **Isometric Exercise for Blood Pressure Control:** Research has shown that isometric exercises, particularly handgrip exercises and static holds like wall sits, can have a significant positive effect on reducing blood pressure. These exercises allow for prolonged muscle tension without dramatically increasing the heart rate. By engaging muscles in a controlled and sustained manner, isometric exercises encourage better blood flow, improve vascular health, and promote more efficient circulation. For individuals with high blood pressure, this means engaging in safe, heart-healthy activities that don't spike blood pressure levels, which can sometimes happen with high-intensity dynamic workouts.

- **Other Types of Exercise:** While aerobic exercises like jogging, swimming, or cycling are also effective for improving cardiovascular health, they often cause a temporary spike in heart rate and blood pressure during intense activity. For individuals with hypertension, this can be concerning, as the goal is to avoid sudden spikes in blood pressure. However, dynamic exercises are still beneficial, as they help with overall heart health and endurance. But they may need to be approached with caution and medical advice for those with severe hypertension.

For individuals looking to control high blood pressure through exercise, isometric training provides a safer, controlled alternative that delivers benefits without increasing the risk of cardiovascular stress.

4. Muscle Engagement and Focus

The way muscles are engaged also sets isometric exercise apart from traditional dynamic exercises.

- **Focused Muscle Engagement in Isometric Exercise:** In isometric exercises, the focus is on **targeted muscle engagement** without movement. This requires the individual to hold a position and actively squeeze or contract the muscle group involved. For example, during a plank, the core, shoulders, and glutes are engaged to keep the body stable. There is a heightened sense of muscle awareness, as you can feel the tension build up during the hold, and it requires concentration and endurance to maintain the position. This can lead to improvements in muscle tone and strength in specific areas, making it a great option for those looking to work on stability or postural strength.

- **Other Types of Exercise:** Dynamic exercises, on the other hand, involve multiple muscle groups in more fluid movements. In activities like running, squatting, or rowing, the muscles are moving through a range of motion. While this improves overall fitness and muscle coordination, it does not target muscles as directly or with the same intensity of focus as isometric exercises do.

If your goal is to improve stability, strengthen specific muscle groups, or focus on endurance, isometric exercises are particularly effective, as they hone in on isolated muscle engagement.

5. Time Efficiency

Isometric exercises are also known for their time efficiency compared to other forms of exercise.

- **Isometric Exercise:** One of the key advantages of isometric exercises is that they require less time to perform while still delivering noticeable results in muscle strength and endurance. Holding a plank or wall sit for 30-60 seconds can engage your muscles in a way that would otherwise take several minutes of dynamic movements to achieve. This makes isometric training ideal for people with busy schedules or those who need quick, effective workouts.

- **Other Types of Exercise:** Dynamic exercises generally take longer to provide the same benefits because they involve multiple repetitions and sets. For example, you may need to perform several sets of squats to feel the same burn you'd get from holding an isometric squat for a shorter period of time. While both forms of exercise are effective, isometric training offers the benefit of efficiency, allowing for shorter workout times with targeted results.

Isometric exercise offers a range of benefits that make it an appealing option for individuals of all fitness levels, especially those managing high blood pressure. While many people are familiar with traditional forms of exercise, such as aerobic activities and weight training, isometric exercises stand out due to their simplicity, efficiency, and low-impact nature. Here's an in-depth look at the key benefits that make isometric exercise such a valuable tool for improving overall health and well-being.

1. Lowering Blood Pressure

One of the most significant benefits of isometric exercise, particularly for individuals with hypertension, is its proven ability to lower blood pressure. Several studies have shown that regular isometric training can lead to reductions in both systolic and diastolic blood pressure. The exact mechanism isn't entirely understood, but it's believed that the sustained muscle contractions during isometric exercises promote better blood flow, improved vascular function, and a reduction in overall cardiovascular strain.

For people who have high blood pressure, finding exercises that don't cause sudden spikes in heart rate or blood pressure is crucial. Isometric exercises allow for slow, controlled movements that keep the heart rate steady, making them a safe and effective option. Over time, consistent engagement in isometric exercises can contribute to healthier blood pressure levels, potentially reducing the need for medication or enhancing the effects of other lifestyle changes like diet and weight management.

2. Improving Muscle Strength and Endurance

Isometric exercises are an excellent way to build both muscle strength and endurance. By holding static positions, such as planks or wall sits, muscles are engaged for an extended period. This sustained contraction forces the muscles to work hard, even though there's no visible movement. Over time, this leads to increased muscle strength as well as greater endurance.

Unlike traditional weightlifting, which requires repetitive movements, isometric exercises focus on maintaining tension, which targets both large and small muscle groups. This can lead to improved muscle tone and the development of stabilizing muscles that support overall movement and posture. Additionally, because you're holding positions for an extended period, your muscles learn to endure sustained tension, improving their overall endurance.

3. Low Impact on Joints

For people with joint pain, arthritis, or those recovering from an injury, isometric exercises provide a low-impact alternative to traditional forms of exercise. Many types of dynamic exercises, such as running or jumping, put stress on the joints, leading to discomfort or even injury. Isometric exercises, on the other hand, require no joint movement, significantly reducing the risk of joint strain.

By engaging the muscles without moving the joints, isometric exercises allow individuals to build strength in a controlled and safe manner. This makes it an ideal form of exercise for people with joint issues or those who are looking for gentle, joint-friendly workouts. Even those with more severe mobility issues can often perform isometric exercises safely, as they can be adapted to individual capabilities.

4. Time-Efficient and Accessible

One of the great advantages of isometric exercises is how efficient and accessible they are. You don't need any special equipment or even a lot of space to perform them. Most isometric exercises, such as planks, wall sits, or handgrip squeezes, can be done anywhere—in your living room, at the office, or even during a break at work. This convenience makes it easier to stay consistent with your workout routine, which is key to achieving long-term health benefits.

Isometric exercises are also quick. A single session may only require holding a position for 10 to 30 seconds, but because the muscles are engaged intensely during that time, the results can be just as effective as longer, more intense workouts. This is a huge benefit for individuals with busy schedules who want to stay fit but may not have time for lengthy workout sessions.

5. Enhanced Core Stability and Posture

Many isometric exercises, such as the plank or wall sit, engage the core muscles, which are essential for maintaining balance, stability, and good posture. By regularly performing isometric exercises that focus on core stability, you strengthen the muscles that support your spine and improve overall body alignment.

Good posture is critical not only for preventing back and neck pain but also for overall functional movement. When your core muscles are strong, you are better able to maintain proper posture throughout the day, whether sitting at a desk or lifting heavy objects. This leads to reduced discomfort, better breathing, and improved body mechanics in everyday activities.

6. Mental Focus and Discipline

One of the more underrated benefits of isometric exercises is the mental discipline they foster. Holding a static position for an extended period requires concentration and focus. You must be mindful of your body's alignment, muscle engagement, and breathing patterns. This focus on staying present during the exercise can serve as a form of mental training, similar to meditation or mindfulness practices.

Developing this level of mental discipline can have positive effects that extend beyond physical fitness. It can help reduce stress, improve mental clarity, and increase your ability to handle discomfort or challenging situations with greater resilience. The sense of control you develop through isometric training can also support other aspects of your life, from work productivity to managing anxiety.

7. Increased Flexibility and Muscle Control

Although isometric exercises don't involve dynamic movement, they can still help improve flexibility and overall muscle control. By holding certain positions, such as a deep squat or lunge, you are engaging the muscles in a controlled manner, which can gradually increase flexibility over time. The constant tension placed on the muscles can lead to improved muscle elasticity and joint mobility.

In addition, isometric exercises enhance proprioception—your awareness of where your body is in space. This improved muscle control and body awareness can help prevent injuries, enhance athletic performance, and improve coordination in everyday activities.

8. Adaptable for All Fitness Levels

Isometric exercises are incredibly versatile and can be adapted to suit any fitness level. Whether you are a beginner or an advanced athlete, you can modify the intensity of an isometric exercise simply by adjusting the length of time you hold a position or increasing the resistance. For beginners, starting with shorter hold times and gradually increasing as strength and endurance build is an easy way to progress without overwhelming the body.

For those more advanced, adding weights or resistance bands to isometric exercises can increase the challenge and lead to even greater strength gains. This adaptability makes isometric exercises a great choice for people of all ages and fitness backgrounds, as they can be tailored to individual needs and goals.

9. Aids in Rehabilitation and Injury Prevention

Isometric exercises are commonly used in rehabilitation programs to help individuals recover from injuries or surgery. Because these exercises don't involve joint movement, they can strengthen muscles without putting additional strain on injured areas. By isolating and engaging specific muscle groups, individuals can rebuild strength and stability in a controlled environment, reducing the risk of re-injury.

Additionally, isometric exercises help improve muscle balance and coordination, which can prevent future injuries. For example, weak core or stabilizing muscles often lead to imbalances that can cause injury during dynamic activities. Isometric training can address these weaknesses and improve muscle symmetry, supporting safer and more effective movement patterns.

10. Supports Cardiovascular Health

While isometric exercises are not typically associated with aerobic fitness, they still offer cardiovascular benefits. By improving muscle efficiency and endurance, isometric exercises contribute to overall heart health. The increased muscle strength leads to improved circulation, better oxygen delivery to tissues, and a reduction in the workload on the heart during everyday activities.

In the context of blood pressure management, isometric exercises have been shown to help regulate heart rate and reduce the strain on the cardiovascular system. For individuals with hypertension, this makes isometric training an effective and safe way to engage in physical activity without causing dangerous spikes in blood pressure.

CHAPTER 2

Understanding High Blood Pressure

What Is High Blood Pressure (Hypertension)

High blood pressure, also known as hypertension, is a medical condition where the force of the blood against the walls of the arteries is consistently too high. Blood pressure is measured by two numbers: systolic and diastolic pressure. The systolic number represents the pressure in your blood vessels when your heart beats, while the diastolic number reflects the pressure when your heart is at rest between beats. Hypertension occurs when these numbers exceed healthy levels, usually above 130/80 mmHg, depending on guidelines.

The danger of hypertension lies in its ability to silently damage the body over time. Often referred to as a "silent killer," high blood pressure frequently has no noticeable symptoms, meaning many individuals are unaware they have the condition until significant damage has occurred. Left untreated, hypertension can lead to severe health issues such as heart disease, stroke, kidney failure, and other life-threatening conditions.

How High Blood Pressure Affects the Body

Hypertension forces the heart to work harder to pump blood throughout the body, putting excessive strain on the heart and arteries. Over time, this extra strain can cause the arteries to thicken, become less flexible, and narrow, reducing blood flow. This process increases the risk of heart attack, stroke, and aneurysm. Additionally, the kidneys, brain, and eyes can also suffer damage from prolonged high blood pressure, leading to kidney disease, cognitive decline, and vision problems.

The Link Between Hypertension and Physical Activity

Physical inactivity is another significant risk factor for high blood pressure. A sedentary lifestyle can lead to weight gain, increased heart strain, and higher blood pressure levels. However, engaging in regular physical activity, particularly aerobic exercise and resistance training, can help lower blood pressure and improve overall cardiovascular health.

Isometric exercise, a less commonly discussed but highly effective form of physical activity, has emerged as a promising way to help manage and reduce hypertension. Unlike traditional forms of exercise, isometric exercises involve holding a static position, engaging muscles without movement. Research has shown that these exercises, when performed consistently, can lead to significant reductions in both systolic and diastolic blood pressure, making them an ideal addition to a hypertension management plan.

Hypertension, or high blood pressure, is a common yet serious condition that can lead to a range of health complications, including heart disease, stroke, and kidney failure. While it often develops without noticeable symptoms, understanding its causes and risk factors is crucial for prevention and management. When combined with an effective intervention like isometric exercise, managing these risk factors becomes even more essential in lowering blood pressure levels. In this section, we explore the primary causes and risk factors of hypertension, which are essential for anyone seeking to improve their cardiovascular health, particularly through isometric exercise.

1. Genetics and Family History

A strong genetic component often influences hypertension. If close family members, such as parents or siblings, have high blood pressure, you are more likely to develop the condition yourself. While you can't control your genetics, knowing your family history can help you stay proactive about prevention. By incorporating lifestyle changes, such as regular isometric exercise, you can potentially mitigate the genetic risk by lowering blood pressure and improving overall heart health.

2. Age

The risk of developing hypertension tends to occur as we age. This is because blood vessels naturally lose some of their elasticity over time, making it harder for blood to flow smoothly. The arteries may stiffen, forcing the heart to work harder to pump blood, which in turn raises blood pressure. While age is an uncontrollable factor, exercise—especially low-impact forms like isometric exercises—can play a significant role in keeping blood pressure in check and maintaining vascular health.

3. Poor Diet and High Sodium Intake

Diet is one of the most modifiable risk factors for hypertension. A diet high in sodium is a primary culprit in raising blood pressure levels. Sodium causes the body to retain water, which increases the volume of blood in the arteries, placing extra pressure on the blood vessel walls. Processed foods, fast foods, and salty snacks are often loaded with hidden sodium, contributing to elevated blood pressure.

Conversely, diets rich in potassium, magnesium, and calcium—nutrients that can help regulate blood pressure—can offset the effects of sodium. When combined with isometric exercises, a balanced diet that emphasizes whole, unprocessed foods can significantly reduce the risk of hypertension.

4. Physical Inactivity

A sedentary lifestyle is a major risk factor for developing hypertension. Physical inactivity leads to poor circulation, increased body weight, and a higher risk of cardiovascular problems. When muscles aren't used regularly, they weaken, and the heart has to work harder to pump blood throughout the body. This increased workload often results in higher blood pressure.

Isometric exercises, which involve holding static positions and engaging muscles without movement, offer a powerful solution for individuals who may struggle with more dynamic or strenuous forms of exercise. Regular engagement in isometric training not only strengthens muscles but also improves vascular function, reducing overall blood pressure levels.

5. Obesity and Weight Gain

Being overweight or obese places additional strain on the heart and increases the risk of developing hypertension. Extra body weight, particularly around the abdomen, can lead to increased insulin resistance, inflammation, and hormonal imbalances—all of which contribute to high blood pressure. Fat tissue also requires more blood supply, meaning that the heart must pump more blood to meet the body's needs, further elevating blood pressure.

By integrating isometric exercise into a weight management plan, individuals can improve muscle tone and strength without putting excessive strain on the joints, making it an excellent exercise option for those who may have mobility or weight-related issues. Reducing body weight, even by a small percentage, can have a significant impact on lowering blood pressure.

6. Excessive Alcohol Consumption

Increase in blood pressure can be as a result of drinking too much of Alcohol. Over time, heavy alcohol consumption can damage the heart, liver, and kidneys, all of which play roles in regulating blood pressure. Alcohol is also calorie-dense, contributing to weight gain, which further increases hypertension risk. Reducing or eliminating alcohol intake can result in noticeable improvements in blood pressure control.

When combined with regular isometric exercise, which supports cardiovascular health without overstressing the heart, cutting back on alcohol can contribute to healthier blood pressure levels.

7. Smoking and Tobacco Use

Smoking is a significant risk factor for high blood pressure. The chemicals in tobacco can damage the lining of the arteries, causing them to narrow and harden, which forces the heart to work harder to pump blood through them. This leads to higher blood pressure and a greater risk of developing heart disease and stroke.

Even exposure to secondhand smoke can contribute to high blood pressure. While quitting smoking is the most effective way to lower this risk, pairing it with cardiovascular-friendly activities like isometric exercise can further improve heart health and reduce blood pressure.

8. Stress and Mental Health

Chronic stress can contribute to hypertension by triggering the release of hormones like cortisol and adrenaline, which cause the heart to beat faster and blood vessels to constrict. This response elevates blood pressure, and when stress becomes a constant part of daily life, it can lead to long-term hypertension. Additionally, individuals who experience high levels of stress may engage in unhealthy coping mechanisms, such as overeating, smoking, or alcohol consumption, which further raise blood pressure.

Incorporating stress-reducing techniques, including mindfulness, meditation, and isometric exercises, can help regulate the body's response to stress. Isometric exercises, in particular, are excellent for mental focus and discipline, providing a calming effect that may help mitigate the impact of stress on blood pressure.

9. Chronic Conditions

Certain chronic conditions, such as diabetes, kidney disease, and sleep apnea, can increase the risk of developing hypertension. For instance, diabetes and hypertension often go hand in hand, as high blood sugar levels can damage the arteries and lead to increased pressure. Kidney disease, meanwhile, affects the body's ability to regulate fluid levels, which can also raise blood pressure. Sleep apnea disrupts breathing during sleep, leading to poor oxygenation and increased strain on the cardiovascular system.

For individuals managing chronic conditions, isometric exercises offer a low-impact, accessible form of physical activity that can help improve cardiovascular health without exacerbating symptoms. Regular engagement in isometric training can contribute to better blood pressure control and overall health outcomes for those dealing with these underlying conditions.

10. Gender and Hormonal Changes

Gender can also play a role in hypertension risk. Before menopause, women tend to have a lower risk of high blood pressure compared to men, but this changes after menopause. The decline in estrogen levels is believed to contribute to a higher risk of hypertension in older women. Additionally, conditions like polycystic ovary syndrome (PCOS) and pregnancy-related complications, such as preeclampsia, can also raise the risk of hypertension in women.

Isometric exercises provide an accessible way for both men and women to manage blood pressure at various stages of life. By maintaining muscle strength and improving vascular health, these exercises can support overall cardiovascular function, regardless of hormonal changes.

Understanding the causes and risk factors of hypertension is crucial for anyone looking to prevent or manage the condition, particularly through lifestyle changes.

High blood pressure, or hypertension, is often called the "silent killer" because it typically shows no symptoms until serious health complications arise. When left untreated, high blood pressure can significantly impact the body, leading to severe and life-threatening conditions. Understanding the health risks associated with untreated hypertension is critical, particularly when considering the role that isometric exercises can play in managing this condition.

1. Heart Disease

One of the most serious consequences of untreated high blood pressure is the increased risk of heart disease. The heart must work harder to pump blood throughout the body when hypertensive. Over time, this added strain can weaken the heart muscle, leading to conditions such as heart failure, coronary artery disease, and an enlarged heart. Untreated high blood pressure can also cause damage to the arteries, leading to atherosclerosis—a buildup of plaque in the arteries—which further increases the risk of heart attacks and strokes.

As hypertension remains untreated, the continuous strain on the cardiovascular system makes it more difficult for blood to flow freely, putting you at greater risk of suffering from cardiovascular events. Isometric exercise is important in this aspects. By helping to reduce blood pressure, isometric exercises can alleviate some of the stress on the heart and blood vessels, promoting cardiovascular health and reducing the risk of heart disease.

2. Stroke

When the brain's blood supply is cut off or diminished, brain tissue is deprived of oxygen and nutrients, leading to a stroke. High blood pressure is the leading cause of strokes because it can weaken blood vessels in the brain, making them more prone to bursting (hemorrhagic stroke) or forming clots (ischemic stroke). Over time, untreated high blood pressure increases the likelihood of these dangerous events, which can result in permanent disability, brain damage, or death.

The ability of isometric exercises to lower blood pressure may help reduce the likelihood of a stroke by improving vascular function and decreasing overall stress on the blood vessels. For individuals at risk of strokes, adopting a routine of isometric exercises could be a preventive measure that supports long-term brain and cardiovascular health.

3. Kidney Damage

The kidneys play a crucial role in filtering waste from the blood and maintaining the body's fluid balance. Damage to the kidneys' blood arteries due to high blood pressure might impair the kidneys' capacity to function normally. This condition, known as hypertensive nephropathy, can lead to chronic kidney disease or kidney failure if left untreated. When the kidneys are unable to efficiently filter waste from the bloodstream, toxins accumulate in the body, which can cause further health complications.

Untreated hypertension is a major cause of end-stage kidney disease, often requiring dialysis or a kidney transplant to manage. Isometric exercises, by helping to lower blood pressure, can be an essential part of preventing kidney damage in individuals with hypertension. While exercise cannot reverse kidney damage, it can prevent further deterioration by promoting better blood pressure control.

4. Vision Loss

High blood pressure can also have a negative impact on vision. The small, delicate blood vessels in the eyes are particularly susceptible to damage from untreated hypertension. Over time, high blood pressure can cause retinopathy, a condition where the blood vessels in the retina (the light-sensitive part of the eye) become damaged. This can lead to blurred vision, bleeding in the eye, and, in severe cases, permanent vision loss.

Additionally, untreated hypertension increases the risk of glaucoma, a condition caused by increased pressure in the eye, which can lead to blindness. By managing blood pressure through isometric exercises, individuals may reduce their risk of developing these vision problems and protect their eye health.

5. Aneurysms

An aneurysm occurs when a weakened section of an artery wall bulges outward, creating a balloon-like appearance. High blood pressure can contribute to the formation of aneurysms by putting excessive force on the arterial walls. Over time, the continuous pressure can cause the weakened artery to rupture, leading to internal bleeding. A ruptured aneurysm is a life-threatening emergency and often results in severe complications or death.

Common sites for aneurysms include the brain, aorta (the largest artery in the body), and abdominal region. The risk of developing an aneurysm increases when high blood pressure is left untreated for extended periods. By helping to lower blood pressure, isometric exercises can reduce the risk of aneurysm formation, providing long-term protection against this potentially fatal condition.

6. Sexual Dysfunction

Hypertension can also lead to sexual dysfunction in both men and women. In men, high blood pressure can cause erectile dysfunction by limiting blood flow to the penis. In women, high blood pressure can reduce blood flow to the reproductive organs, leading to decreased sexual arousal, lubrication issues, and overall satisfaction. The reduced blood flow caused by untreated hypertension makes it difficult for individuals to maintain healthy sexual function, which can have significant effects on quality of life and relationships.

By lowering blood pressure through isometric exercise, individuals can improve circulation, which may help prevent sexual dysfunction related to hypertension. Improved vascular health means better blood flow, potentially enhancing sexual function and contributing to better overall well-being.

7. Cognitive Decline

Untreated high blood pressure can also lead to cognitive decline and an increased risk of dementia. Chronic hypertension reduces the flow of blood to the brain, which can impair memory, cognitive functions, and the ability to learn or make decisions. Over time, untreated hypertension may lead to conditions such as vascular dementia, where cognitive decline results from reduced blood supply to brain tissues.

Maintaining healthy blood pressure levels through isometric exercises may protect against cognitive decline by improving blood flow to the brain and ensuring that brain cells receive the oxygen and nutrients they need. Regular exercise, including isometric activities, can promote mental clarity, enhance memory, and support long-term brain health.

8. Peripheral Artery Disease (PAD)

Peripheral artery disease occurs when plaque builds up in the arteries that supply blood to the limbs, particularly the legs. High blood pressure accelerates the hardening of the arteries (atherosclerosis), which can reduce blood flow to the legs and feet. PAD often causes pain, cramping, numbness, or weakness in the legs, especially during physical activity. If left untreated, PAD can lead to serious complications such as infections, tissue death, or the need for amputation.

Isometric exercises can help improve circulation and blood vessel function, reducing the risk of PAD. While these exercises focus on muscle contractions without movement, they still engage the cardiovascular system, helping to promote better blood flow and prevent the progression of peripheral artery disease.

9. Weakened Immune System

High blood pressure can weaken the immune system, making it harder for the body to fight off infections and diseases. Chronic hypertension puts stress on the body, increasing inflammation and reducing the body's ability to respond to illness. Untreated high blood pressure may lead to frequent illnesses, slower recovery times, and increased susceptibility to infections such as colds, flu, and more serious conditions.

By lowering blood pressure through isometric exercise, individuals can support their immune function and improve their body's ability to defend itself against infections. A well-functioning immune system is vital for overall health and longevity, making blood pressure management an essential part of maintaining a strong immune response.

10. Shortened Life Expectancy

Perhaps one of the most sobering risks of untreated high blood pressure is its effect on life expectancy. Hypertension significantly increases the risk of heart disease, stroke, kidney failure, and other life-threatening conditions, all of which can shorten life expectancy. Studies have shown that individuals with untreated hypertension have a higher risk of premature death compared to those who manage their blood pressure effectively.

Incorporating isometric exercises as part of a comprehensive blood pressure management plan can help reduce the risk of these serious complications, potentially extending lifespan and improving overall quality of life. Maintaining healthy blood pressure is key to longevity and preventing the numerous health risks associated with untreated hypertension.

CHAPTER 3

The Connection Between Isometric Exercise and Blood Pressure

How Isometric Exercise Helps Lower Blood Pressure

Isometric exercise has gained attention as a powerful tool for managing and reducing high blood pressure, or hypertension, in a safe and effective way. Unlike aerobic exercises or high-intensity workouts, isometric exercises involve static muscle contractions without movement, making them an excellent option for those with cardiovascular concerns. But how exactly does isometric exercise help lower blood pressure? Here's an extensive look at the mechanisms and benefits behind it.

1. Vascular Adaptations

One of the primary ways isometric exercise helps lower blood pressure is through vascular adaptations. When you perform isometric exercises, the muscles contract and maintain tension over a period of time, causing blood vessels to constrict. During this process, the muscles demand more oxygen, and the heart works to deliver blood to the muscles under tension. Over time, this repeated constriction and relaxation of blood vessels improves their elasticity, making them more adaptable to changes in blood flow.

As a result, the blood vessels become more efficient at regulating blood pressure, allowing them to dilate more easily when necessary. This improved vascular function reduces the overall strain on the heart and helps regulate blood pressure levels, particularly in individuals with hypertension. Essentially, isometric exercise "trains" the blood vessels to handle pressure fluctuations more effectively.

2. Reduction in Sympathetic Nervous System Activity

The sympathetic nervous system (SNS) is responsible for the body's "fight or flight" response, which includes increasing heart rate and constricting blood vessels. In people with high blood pressure, the SNS tends to be overactive, leading to elevated heart rate and vasoconstriction (narrowing of blood vessels), which in turn raises blood pressure.

Isometric exercises have been shown to reduce the activity of the sympathetic nervous system, which directly impacts blood pressure. By lowering the SNS response, isometric exercises help to relax blood vessels and decrease heart rate, reducing the overall pressure in the circulatory system. This decrease in SNS activity creates a calming effect on the cardiovascular system, leading to more stable and lower blood pressure readings over time.

3. Enhanced Baroreflex Sensitivity

The baroreflex is a critical mechanism in the body that helps regulate blood pressure. It acts as a feedback loop between the heart and the brain, constantly monitoring and adjusting blood pressure in response to changes in body position or activity. In people with high blood pressure, the baroreflex is often impaired, making it less effective at maintaining stable blood pressure levels.

Research indicates that regular isometric exercise can enhance baroreflex sensitivity, improving the body's ability to regulate blood pressure. By strengthening the connection between the cardiovascular system and the brain, isometric exercises make the baroreflex more responsive, allowing it to better adjust to shifts in blood pressure. This means that individuals who regularly perform isometric exercises are likely to experience fewer sudden increases in blood pressure during daily activities, helping to maintain a healthier baseline.

4. Reduction of Peripheral Resistance

Peripheral resistance refers to the resistance that blood vessels offer to the flow of blood. High blood pressure often occurs when the arteries become narrow, stiff, or blocked, making it harder for blood to flow smoothly. This increased resistance forces the heart to work harder to pump blood through the body, elevating blood pressure.

Isometric exercises can help reduce peripheral resistance by promoting vasodilation, or the widening of blood vessels. When the muscles contract during isometric exercises, they temporarily restrict blood flow. Once the contraction is released, blood flow returns, and the blood vessels naturally dilate. Regularly practicing this pattern of contraction and relaxation helps the blood vessels become more flexible, reducing overall resistance in the circulatory system. This reduction in peripheral resistance translates into lower blood pressure, as the heart no longer has to pump as forcefully to circulate blood.

5. Improved Endothelial Function

The thin layer of cells lining the inside of blood vessels is called the endothelium. It plays a crucial role in maintaining vascular health by regulating blood flow and releasing substances that control blood clotting, immune function, and vascular relaxation. Poor endothelial function is often associated with hypertension, as it impairs the ability of blood vessels to expand and contract effectively.

Isometric exercise has been found to improve endothelial function, making blood vessels more responsive to changes in blood pressure. During isometric exercises, the endothelium is stimulated, promoting the release of nitric oxide—a molecule that causes blood vessels to relax and dilate. This improved endothelial function not only helps lower blood pressure but also contributes to overall cardiovascular health by reducing the risk of atherosclerosis (hardening of the arteries) and other related conditions.

6. Increased Parasympathetic Nervous System Activity

While isometric exercise reduces the activity of the sympathetic nervous system, it simultaneously enhances the activity of the parasympathetic nervous system (PNS), often referred to as the "rest and digest" system. The PNS plays an essential role in counterbalancing the effects of the SNS by slowing down the heart rate and promoting relaxation throughout the body.

Regular engagement in isometric exercises helps stimulate the PNS, which in turn leads to lower blood pressure. As the parasympathetic nervous system becomes more dominant, the body experiences less stress and tension, further contributing to better cardiovascular regulation and lower resting blood pressure levels. This increase in parasympathetic activity also helps individuals manage stress more effectively, which is a common trigger for blood pressure spikes.

7. Hormonal Balance and Reduced Stress

Chronic stress is a well-known contributor to high blood pressure. When the body is under stress, it releases hormones like cortisol and adrenaline, which can cause blood pressure to rise. Isometric exercise has been shown to reduce levels of stress hormones, helping to create a more balanced hormonal environment. By lowering the levels of these hormones, isometric exercises help prevent stress-induced blood pressure spikes, making it easier to manage hypertension in the long term.

Additionally, isometric exercise promotes the release of endorphins, often called "feel-good" hormones, which help improve mood and reduce feelings of stress and anxiety. This hormonal shift creates a more relaxed state, which can help lower blood pressure during both exercise and rest.

8. Improved Heart Efficiency

Isometric exercise helps improve heart efficiency by strengthening the heart muscle without significantly increasing heart rate. Unlike aerobic exercises that cause the heart to beat faster to meet the oxygen demands of the body, isometric exercises promote strength without putting excessive strain on the heart. This leads to a more efficient heart that can pump blood with less effort, thereby reducing the force needed to circulate blood throughout the body.

For individuals with high blood pressure, this improved heart efficiency can lead to a decrease in overall cardiovascular strain, allowing the heart to maintain healthy blood pressure levels with less exertion.

9. Adaptability to Different Fitness Levels

One of the unique advantages of isometric exercises is their adaptability, which makes them accessible to individuals at various fitness levels, including those with high blood pressure. Since isometric exercises can be modified to suit the individual's abilities and needs, they are a safe and effective option for people with hypertension who may be concerned about engaging in high-intensity workouts that could spike blood pressure.

The low-impact nature of isometric exercises ensures that individuals can perform them without excessive stress on the cardiovascular system, providing a controlled environment for gradual blood pressure reduction.

By integrating isometric exercises into a daily or weekly routine, individuals with hypertension can achieve significant improvements in blood pressure regulation, cardiovascular health, and overall well-being. The simplicity, safety, and effectiveness of these exercises make them a valuable component of any blood pressure management plan.

The Role of Muscle Contraction in Cardiovascular Health

Muscle contraction plays a crucial role in cardiovascular health, particularly in the context of isometric exercise for managing high blood pressure. Understanding how muscles interact with the cardiovascular system during contraction can provide insights into how isometric exercises help regulate blood pressure and improve overall heart health. Unlike dynamic exercises, where muscles undergo repeated cycles of contraction and relaxation, isometric exercises involve sustained muscle contractions without joint movement. This unique aspect of isometric exercise can have profound effects on cardiovascular function.

1. Improved Blood Flow and Circulation

When muscles contract during isometric exercises, they exert pressure on the blood vessels within and around them. This pressure temporarily reduces blood flow to the working muscles, prompting the heart to work harder to maintain circulation. However, upon relaxation, the blood vessels dilate, allowing for an increased rush of blood back into the muscles. This process enhances blood flow and improves circulation throughout the body.

By regularly engaging in isometric exercises, individuals can promote better vascular health. The periodic constriction and dilation of blood vessels help improve their elasticity, which is vital for maintaining healthy blood pressure levels. More elastic blood vessels can expand and contract more efficiently, reducing the overall workload on the heart and lowering the risk of hypertension.

2. Increased Vascular Resistance and Blood Pressure Regulation

The sustained muscle contractions in isometric exercises lead to increased vascular resistance, a key factor in regulating blood pressure. During isometric exercises, the body experiences a temporary rise in both systolic and diastolic blood pressure. However, this increase is typically followed by a longer-term reduction in resting blood pressure after the exercise is completed. This phenomenon is particularly beneficial for individuals with high blood pressure, as regular isometric training can result in more stable blood pressure levels over time.

One of the reasons for this improvement is that isometric exercises enhance the strength of the blood vessels, making them more capable of handling fluctuations in pressure. This strengthens the cardiovascular system's ability to regulate blood pressure during both periods of activity and rest. The ability of isometric exercise to improve vascular resistance and blood pressure regulation makes it a valuable tool for managing hypertension without placing undue stress on the heart.

3. Reduced Workload on the Heart

Muscle contraction during isometric exercises can help reduce the overall workload on the heart. The heart's primary job is to pump oxygen-rich blood to the body's tissues, and this task becomes more challenging when blood vessels are stiff or blocked. However, regular isometric training helps to improve the efficiency of the heart by increasing the strength of the muscles and promoting better vascular function.

As the muscles become stronger, they require less effort from the heart to deliver blood to them during both rest and activity. This means that over time, the heart does not need to work as hard to circulate blood, reducing the risk of heart-related complications such as hypertensive heart disease or heart failure. By reducing the heart's workload, isometric exercises help ensure that the cardiovascular system operates more efficiently, which is essential for individuals managing high blood pressure.

4. Enhanced Oxygen Delivery to Tissues

Another critical aspect of muscle contraction's role in cardiovascular health is the improved oxygen delivery to tissues. When muscles contract, they demand more oxygen to fuel the effort. The cardiovascular system responds by increasing blood flow to the muscles, ensuring that oxygen is delivered where it's needed most. With repeated isometric training, the body becomes more efficient at oxygen delivery, improving both cardiovascular function and muscle endurance.

This enhanced oxygen delivery helps reduce the strain on the cardiovascular system, particularly during physical activity. The improved oxygenation of muscles and tissues leads to better overall health and reduced fatigue, allowing individuals to perform everyday tasks with greater ease. For those with high blood pressure, this means that the body can manage physical exertion more efficiently, further aiding in the regulation of blood pressure levels.

5. Activation of the Parasympathetic Nervous System

Sustained muscle contractions during isometric exercises can also stimulate the parasympathetic nervous system, which is responsible for the body's "rest and digest" response. The parasympathetic nervous system helps counteract the "fight or flight" response associated with stress and high blood pressure. By engaging in isometric exercises, individuals can activate this system, leading to a calming effect on the cardiovascular system.

The parasympathetic response lowers heart rate and promotes relaxation of the blood vessels, contributing to long-term reductions in blood pressure. This effect is particularly beneficial for people with hypertension, as chronic stress and an overactive sympathetic nervous system can exacerbate high blood pressure. Isometric exercises help balance this response, providing both physical and psychological benefits for cardiovascular health.

6. Improved Endothelial Function

Endothelial cells line the inside of blood vessels and play a key role in vascular health. They regulate blood vessel dilation, control blood flow, and help prevent the buildup of plaque. Muscle contraction during isometric exercise has been shown to improve endothelial function by promoting the release of nitric oxide, a molecule that helps blood vessels relax and widen. Improved endothelial function is crucial for maintaining healthy blood pressure and reducing the risk of cardiovascular disease.

By enhancing the health of the endothelial cells, isometric exercise supports better blood flow and reduces the risk of atherosclerosis—a condition in which the arteries become narrowed due to plaque buildup. For individuals with high blood pressure, maintaining healthy endothelial function is critical in preventing further cardiovascular complications.

7. Cardiovascular Efficiency and Adaptation

Isometric exercises, through muscle contraction, improve overall cardiovascular efficiency. The heart becomes better at pumping blood, and the blood vessels become more responsive to changes in pressure and demand. This increased efficiency allows the cardiovascular system to adapt more easily to the body's needs, both during exercise and rest. Over time, the cardiovascular system becomes more resilient, making it easier to manage blood pressure levels and reduce the risk of hypertension-related complications.

Over the past few decades, a growing body of research has emerged, supporting the efficacy of isometric exercise as a beneficial tool for managing hypertension. While traditional aerobic and resistance training exercises have long been recommended for cardiovascular health, isometric exercise has increasingly gained recognition for its ability to lower blood pressure, particularly for individuals with high blood pressure. Below is an exploration of some of the key studies and findings that highlight the connection between isometric exercise and hypertension management.

1. The British Journal of Sports Medicine Study (2013)

A landmark study published in the *British Journal of Sports Medicine* in 2013 brought significant attention to the role of isometric exercise in reducing blood pressure. This meta-analysis reviewed multiple studies that examined the effects of isometric resistance training on blood pressure and found that isometric exercises, such as handgrip training, significantly lowered both systolic and diastolic blood pressure in participants. The reductions averaged about 10 mmHg for systolic and 7 mmHg for diastolic blood pressure—figures comparable to, or even better than, the results seen from aerobic exercise programs.

The researchers suggested that the reduction in blood pressure could be attributed to improved vascular function, including enhanced endothelial function (the health of the lining of blood vessels) and a decrease in peripheral resistance. This study was pivotal in establishing isometric exercise as a non-pharmacological intervention for managing hypertension.

2. Canadian Study on Isometric Handgrip Training (2010)

Another significant study conducted by the *Canadian Journal of Cardiology* in 2010 examined the effects of isometric handgrip exercises on individuals with hypertension. The research involved participants performing handgrip exercises several times a week over a 10-week period. The results were notable: systolic blood pressure was reduced by an average of 15 mmHg, and diastolic blood pressure was reduced by 6 mmHg.

The study concluded that isometric handgrip exercises were effective in lowering blood pressure, especially for those who were not engaging in other forms of physical activity. The researchers also noted that the exercises were particularly beneficial for individuals who had difficulty performing aerobic activities, such as older adults or those with joint issues.

3. American Heart Association's Endorsement (2017)

The American Heart Association (AHA) has also acknowledged the potential benefits of isometric exercise in managing blood pressure. In its 2017 guidelines, the AHA mentioned isometric handgrip exercises as a promising adjunct to other lifestyle modifications for lowering blood pressure. While the AHA did not yet fully endorse isometric exercises as a primary treatment, it recognized the growing evidence supporting their use as part of a comprehensive approach to hypertension management.

This recognition from a leading cardiovascular authority further solidified isometric exercise's place in the conversation around hypertension treatment. The AHA's endorsement, though measured, indicated that isometric exercise had made significant strides in being considered a viable option for blood pressure control.

4. Mayo Clinic Study (2018)

A study conducted by the Mayo Clinic in 2018 explored the relationship between isometric exercise and blood pressure regulation in both healthy adults and those with elevated blood pressure. The study involved participants completing four sets of isometric handgrip exercises per week over a six-week period. The findings indicated a reduction of up to 13 mmHg in systolic blood pressure for participants with hypertension.

Interestingly, the study also found that the effects of isometric exercise were cumulative. The more consistently the participants engaged in the handgrip exercises, the greater the reduction in blood pressure over time. This suggested that isometric exercises could be integrated into a long-term exercise routine for sustained blood pressure management.

5. University of Exeter Study (2020)

Research conducted at the *University of Exeter* in 2020 delved into the mechanisms behind the blood pressure-lowering effects of isometric exercises. The study involved both young and older adults and examined the physiological changes that occurred during isometric exercise. The findings indicated that isometric exercises led to improved autonomic control of the heart and blood vessels. More specifically, it suggested that isometric training could improve baroreceptor sensitivity—a key factor in the body's ability to regulate blood pressure.

Baroreceptors are sensors in the cardiovascular system that detect changes in blood pressure and help maintain stability. Improved baroreceptor function means that the body can better regulate blood pressure, particularly in response to stress or physical activity. This study provided further insight into how isometric exercises directly influence the cardiovascular system in ways that benefit individuals with hypertension.

6. Journal of Hypertension Review (2019)

A review published in the *Journal of Hypertension* in 2019 evaluated the long-term effects of isometric resistance training on individuals with stage 1 and stage 2 hypertension. The review included over 20 studies involving participants who engaged in various forms of isometric exercises, such as handgrip training, wall sits, and plank holds.

The results were overwhelmingly positive, with many studies showing an average reduction of 10-12 mmHg in systolic blood pressure and 5-8 mmHg in diastolic blood pressure. Additionally, the review highlighted that isometric exercises were particularly effective in lowering blood pressure in individuals who had previously been resistant to other forms of exercise or lifestyle interventions.

The authors of the review noted that isometric exercise had the potential to become a more widely recommended treatment option for hypertension, particularly in populations where traditional exercise regimens were impractical or unsafe.

7. European Society of Hypertension (ESH) Guidelines (2022)

In its 2022 guidelines, the *European Society of Hypertension* incorporated isometric exercise as part of its recommendations for non-pharmacological management of hypertension. The ESH cited several studies, including those mentioned above, that supported the use of isometric resistance training for lowering blood pressure. The society emphasized the role of isometric exercises in improving vascular function and reducing arterial stiffness—two key factors that contribute to hypertension.

The ESH guidelines also pointed out that isometric exercises can be easily integrated into daily routines, making them accessible for a wide range of individuals, including those with limited mobility or those who struggle to adhere to traditional exercise programs. This acknowledgment from a leading international authority further reinforced the credibility of isometric exercise as a practical solution for blood pressure control.

8. Johns Hopkins University Study (2021)

In a 2021 study conducted by *Johns Hopkins University*, researchers explored the long-term effects of isometric exercise on cardiovascular health in adults aged 40 and older. The study found that not only did participants experience significant reductions in blood pressure, but they also saw improvements in arterial flexibility and decreased markers of inflammation.

One of the contributing factors to hypertension is Chronic inflammation and other cardiovascular diseases. The Johns Hopkins study suggested that isometric exercises could reduce inflammation by improving blood vessel function and reducing oxidative stress. These findings were particularly important for older adults, as inflammation and arterial stiffness are often more pronounced in this population.

The study's results indicated that isometric exercises could have a broader range of cardiovascular benefits beyond just blood pressure reduction, making them a valuable tool for improving overall heart health in individuals with hypertension.

9. Handgrip Exercises in Geriatric Populations (2020)

A study published in the *Journal of Geriatric Cardiology* in 2020 focused on the effects of isometric handgrip exercises in older adults with high blood pressure. The study found that participants who engaged in just 15 minutes of handgrip exercises per day, three times a week, experienced significant reductions in blood pressure over a six-month period.

This study was particularly noteworthy because it demonstrated the potential for isometric exercise to be used as a low-risk, high-reward intervention for older adults who may not be able to perform more strenuous physical activity. The researchers concluded that isometric handgrip exercises could be an important part of a comprehensive blood pressure management plan, especially for elderly individuals who face mobility challenges.

CHAPTER 4

Getting Started with Isometric Exercise

Who Should Perform Isometric Exercises

Isometric exercises are highly adaptable and accessible, making them suitable for a wide range of individuals. However, when considering isometric exercises in the context of managing high blood pressure, it's important to identify specific groups that could benefit most from this type of exercise. While isometric training is generally safe, certain individuals will find it especially effective for improving their health and fitness without putting undue strain on their cardiovascular system.

1. Individuals with High Blood Pressure (Hypertension)

The primary group who should incorporate isometric exercises into their routine are those who have been diagnosed with high blood pressure. Research has consistently shown that isometric exercise can reduce both systolic and diastolic blood pressure, making it an excellent non-pharmaceutical approach to managing hypertension. Unlike more intense cardiovascular exercises, which can cause spikes in blood pressure during activity, isometric exercises are performed in a controlled, static manner, preventing dramatic fluctuations in heart rate.

For individuals with hypertension, engaging in physical activity that doesn't overly stress the cardiovascular system is crucial. Isometric exercises fit this need perfectly because they allow the muscles to work without causing the sudden increases in blood pressure that might come with high-intensity aerobic activities. Regular practice can lead to long-term improvements in vascular function, reducing the overall risk of heart disease and stroke.

2. Older Adults

As we age, maintaining muscle strength and joint stability becomes more important, but many older adults are wary of engaging in high-impact or strenuous activities that might lead to injury. Isometric exercises are an ideal solution for this population because they provide a low-impact way to build strength and stability without placing excess stress on the joints or cardiovascular system. Older adults, especially those with hypertension, can use isometric training to improve muscle tone, enhance balance, and prevent the loss of strength that comes with aging.

Furthermore, because isometric exercises do not involve movement, they are safe for individuals with arthritis or joint issues. They can be done while seated or standing, and the intensity can be modified based on the individual's fitness level. This makes it an excellent option for seniors looking to stay active and manage their blood pressure without the risk of injury or overexertion.

3. People with Joint Pain or Arthritis

For individuals suffering from joint pain or arthritis, traditional exercises that require repetitive movement can aggravate their condition. Isometric exercises, on the other hand, involve no joint movement, making them an excellent choice for people with joint issues. Since isometric exercises rely on static muscle contractions, they provide a way to strengthen the muscles around the joints without causing additional wear and tear.

Those with arthritis or chronic joint pain often struggle to find safe exercises that won't exacerbate their symptoms, but isometric exercises allow them to build strength and improve mobility in a pain-free way. For this group, strengthening the muscles that support the joints can lead to better joint stability, improved function, and a reduction in pain over time.

4. Individuals with Limited Mobility

People who have limited mobility due to injury, disability, or chronic conditions like multiple sclerosis can greatly benefit from isometric exercises. Because these exercises do not require large ranges of motion or dynamic movements, they are perfect for individuals who may not be able to perform traditional strength training exercises. Isometric exercises can often be performed while sitting or lying down, making them accessible for individuals with mobility challenges.

Moreover, isometric exercises can help this group maintain muscle mass, improve circulation, and prevent the decline in strength and flexibility that often comes with restricted movement. For those who are wheelchair-bound or recovering from surgery, isometric training offers a safe way to stay physically active and manage blood pressure effectively.

5. Busy Individuals Seeking Time-Efficient Workouts

For people who lead busy lives and struggle to find time for exercise, isometric exercises provide a time-efficient solution. Many isometric exercises can be performed in just a few minutes and don't require any special equipment or gym access. This makes it easy for individuals to fit these exercises into their daily routine, even if they only have a few spare minutes at home or in the office.

The simplicity and efficiency of isometric exercises are perfect for those who may not have time for lengthy workouts but still want to improve their health. And since managing blood pressure often requires consistency, isometric exercises allow individuals to maintain a regular exercise routine without having to commit large amounts of time.

6. People New to Exercise

Isometric exercises are particularly well-suited for individuals who are new to exercise or those who have not been physically active for some time. Unlike more complex exercise programs, isometric exercises are easy to learn and perform, making them an accessible entry point for beginners. There's no need to learn complicated techniques or invest in expensive equipment, as most isometric exercises can be performed using just body weight or simple household items like a wall or chair.

For people who may feel intimidated by traditional exercise routines, isometric exercises offer a way to build strength and improve health in a gentle, manageable way. As a result, they can quickly build confidence and make exercise a regular part of their lives, which is especially important for those looking to manage high blood pressure.

7. Those Looking for Low-Impact Exercise

For individuals who need a low-impact workout, such as people recovering from injury or those with chronic conditions that limit their ability to perform high-impact exercises, isometric exercises offer a safe alternative. The low-impact nature of these exercises ensures that they can be performed without putting stress on the joints, ligaments, or cardiovascular system. This makes them a good choice for individuals who want to strengthen their muscles and improve their health without causing undue strain on their body.

Isometric exercises also allow individuals to increase the intensity at their own pace. This flexibility makes it easy for people to gradually build strength and endurance without risking overexertion or injury.

8. Athletes and Fitness Enthusiasts

Even though isometric exercises are often associated with rehabilitation and gentle workouts, athletes and fitness enthusiasts can also benefit from adding them to their routines. Isometric exercises help improve muscular endurance, core strength, and stability, which are all critical components of athletic performance. Many athletes use isometric training as a way to target smaller, stabilizing muscles that might be neglected during traditional dynamic workouts.

Additionally, for athletes looking to avoid overtraining or injury during intense periods of competition or heavy training, isometric exercises provide a way to maintain muscle engagement without putting additional strain on their bodies. For example, isometric planks, wall sits, and holds can be included in a strength routine to enhance performance while minimizing fatigue and the risk of injury.

9. People Recovering from Surgery or Injury

For individuals recovering from surgery or an injury, traditional exercise may be too strenuous during the early stages of recovery. Isometric exercises offer a gentle way to maintain or rebuild strength while avoiding the risk of re-injury. Because they involve static contractions rather than dynamic movements, these exercises are less likely to cause harm to healing tissues.

Physical therapists often recommend isometric exercises for patients in rehabilitation because they can be performed safely even when full range of motion is not yet possible. By focusing on static holds, individuals can strengthen specific muscle groups that will support their recovery and overall rehabilitation process.

When it comes to incorporating isometric exercises into your routine, especially if you have high blood pressure, prioritizing safety is crucial. While isometric exercises are generally low-impact and accessible, following specific guidelines can help ensure that you exercise safely and effectively. Here are essential safety guidelines and precautions to consider before starting your isometric exercise regimen.

1. Consult with Your Healthcare Provider

Before embarking on any new exercise program, especially if you have a pre-existing medical condition like hypertension, it's vital to consult with your healthcare provider. They can provide personalized recommendations based on your medical history, current health status, and specific needs. This step is particularly important if you're on medication for high blood pressure, as exercise can impact how your body responds to treatment.

2. Start Slowly and Gradually Increase Intensity

It's essential to start slowly if you are new. Begin with shorter holds—around 10 to 15 seconds—and gradually increase the duration as your strength and endurance improve. This gradual approach will help your body adapt without overexerting yourself, which could lead to injury or strain.

3. Focus on Proper Form and Alignment

Maintaining proper form during isometric exercises is crucial for both effectiveness and safety. Poor form can lead to unnecessary strain on your joints and muscles. Take the time to learn the correct positioning for each exercise, ensuring that your body is aligned properly. You may consider working with a physical therapist or a certified trainer who can guide you in executing exercises correctly.

4. Listen to Your Body

Pay attention to how your body responds during and after each exercise session. It's normal to feel muscle fatigue and a burn during isometric holds, but sharp pain or discomfort is a sign that you may be pushing too hard. If you experience any unusual symptoms, such as dizziness, shortness of breath, or chest pain, stop exercising immediately and consult your healthcare provider.

5. Avoid Breath-Holding

One common mistake during isometric exercises is holding your breath while maintaining muscle tension. Breath-holding can cause spikes in blood pressure, which is particularly concerning for individuals with hypertension. Instead, focus on maintaining a steady, controlled breathing pattern throughout each exercise. Inhale deeply as you prepare for the hold, and exhale slowly during the exercise to help keep your blood pressure stable.

6. Choose Appropriate Exercises

Not all isometric exercises are suitable for everyone, especially individuals with high blood pressure. Focus on exercises that promote stability and strength without excessive strain. Avoid positions that put pressure on the head or neck, such as certain variations of planks or push-ups. Exercises like wall sits, seated leg extensions, and handgrip squeezes are generally safer options for those managing hypertension.

7. Stay Hydrated

Staying properly hydrated is essential for overall health and can help maintain stable blood pressure levels. Before, during, and after your exercise sessions, ensure you are drinking enough water. Dehydration can lead to an increase in heart rate and a decrease in performance, so keep a water bottle nearby and take sips as needed.

8. Consider Environmental Factors

When performing isometric exercises, consider your environment. Ensure that the space is free from clutter and hazards to prevent slips or falls. If you're exercising outdoors, choose a comfortable temperature and avoid extreme weather conditions, which can affect your performance and overall well-being.

9. Incorporate Warm-Up and Cool-Down

Before starting your isometric exercises, include a warm-up routine to prepare your muscles and joints. This could involve light stretching or gentle movements to increase blood flow and reduce the risk of injury. Similarly, after completing your workout, take time to cool down and stretch, which can help alleviate muscle tension and promote recovery.

10. Monitor Your Blood Pressure

If you have high blood pressure, consider monitoring your levels before and after exercising. This will help you understand how your body responds to isometric exercises and whether any adjustments are needed in your routine. Use a home blood pressure monitor or consult your healthcare provider for guidance on the best practices for monitoring.

11. Stay Consistent but Flexible

Consistency is essential for seeing the benefits of isometric exercise. However, it's also important to remain flexible with your routine. If you feel fatigued, unwell, or overly stressed, it may be best to skip a session or modify your exercises. Listen to your body and prioritize your health over strict adherence to a schedule.

By following these safety guidelines and precautions, you can safely integrate isometric exercises into your routine, supporting your journey toward managing high blood pressure and improving your overall fitness. The focus should always be on quality over quantity, ensuring that you engage in exercises that promote health and well-being without compromising safety.

While one of the greatest advantages of isometric exercise is that it can often be performed with little to no equipment, certain tools can enhance your training experience, make exercises more effective, and offer greater variety. Here's a detailed look at the recommended equipment for isometric training, particularly in the context of managing high blood pressure and ensuring a safe, effective workout routine.

1. Resistance Bands

Resistance bands are a versatile and affordable option for isometric training. They come in various resistance levels, allowing you to adjust the intensity of your workouts as you progress. Bands can be used for a variety of isometric exercises, such as bicep curls or shoulder presses, where you hold the tension of the band in a fixed position.

Benefits:

- **Portable and Lightweight:** Resistance bands are easy to carry, making them a great option for at-home workouts or for taking to the gym.
- **Customizable Resistance:** You can change the resistance level simply by using bands of different thickness or by adjusting the length of the band.
- **Joint-Friendly:** Bands provide a smooth, gradual resistance that minimizes stress on the joints, which is especially beneficial for individuals with hypertension or joint issues.

2. Stability Balls

Stability balls (also known as exercise or Swiss balls) can be integrated into isometric exercises to enhance core stability and engagement. Holding a position while balancing on a stability ball forces your body to recruit multiple muscle groups, particularly those in the core.

Benefits:

- **Core Engagement:** Using a stability ball helps improve balance and stability while strengthening core muscles, which is essential for good posture and overall functional fitness.
- **Versatile Exercises:** You can perform various isometric exercises, such as wall sits or planks, on a stability ball to increase the challenge and effectiveness of your routine.
- **Promotes Good Posture:** Incorporating stability balls into your workouts can help develop better posture and muscle control.

3. Weighted Vests

Weighted vests can add an extra challenge to your isometric exercises without compromising the integrity of the movements. By increasing your body weight, you can intensify the resistance during static holds, such as wall sits or planks.

Benefits:

- **Progressive Overload:** Adding weight gradually can help you build strength more effectively as you progress in your fitness journey.
- **Enhanced Muscle Activation:** The additional weight forces your muscles to engage more intensely during isometric holds, promoting greater strength gains.
- **Customizable:** Most weighted vests come with adjustable weights, allowing you to tailor the intensity of your workout to your individual fitness level.

4. Foam Rollers

Foam rollers are primarily known for their use in self-myofascial release and recovery, but they can also be utilized for isometric exercises. For example, placing a foam roller between your back and the wall while holding a wall sit can engage your muscles more effectively.

Benefits:

- **Improved Stability:** Using a foam roller can enhance balance and stability during certain isometric exercises, making them more challenging.
- **Injury Prevention:** Regular use of foam rollers aids in muscle recovery and can prevent injuries, ensuring that you remain active and pain-free while managing your blood pressure.
- **Flexibility:** Foam rollers can help improve overall flexibility, which can enhance performance in

various exercises and contribute to better muscle function.

5. Hand Grippers

Hand grippers are a simple yet effective tool for performing isometric exercises targeting the hands and forearms. By squeezing the gripper and holding the contraction, you can strengthen your grip and improve forearm endurance.

Benefits:

- **Focus on Grip Strength:** Hand strength is essential for daily activities and overall functional fitness. Strengthening the hands can enhance your performance in other exercises as well.
- **Portable:** Hand grippers are compact and easy to use anywhere, making them a convenient option for adding isometric training to your routine.
- **Joint-Friendly:** Using hand grippers allows you to engage the muscles without putting stress on the joints, which is important for individuals with high blood pressure or joint concerns.

6. Body Weight

One of the simplest and most effective tools for isometric training is your own body weight. Many isometric exercises can be performed using just your body, such as planks, wall sits, and static lunges. This makes isometric training highly accessible, as no additional equipment is required.

Benefits:

- **No Cost:** Utilizing your body weight eliminates the need for expensive equipment or gym memberships, making isometric training accessible to everyone.
- **Customizable Intensity:** You can easily adjust the intensity of your workout by modifying the duration of holds or the difficulty of the positions.
- **Functional Fitness:** Bodyweight exercises mimic real-life movements and activities, enhancing your functional strength for everyday tasks.

7. Yoga Straps

Yoga straps can be a helpful tool for isometric training, particularly for those looking to improve flexibility and stability. By using a strap, you can hold positions more comfortably and maintain proper alignment during isometric exercises.

Benefits:

- **Assists with Form:** Yoga straps help ensure correct posture and alignment during isometric exercises, reducing the risk of injury and enhancing effectiveness.
- **Flexibility Improvement:** Straps allow you to extend your range of motion, making it easier to hold challenging positions and improve overall flexibility.

- **Adaptability:** They can be used for various exercises, from simple stretches to more complex isometric holds.

8. Exercise Mats

While not a piece of exercise equipment in the traditional sense, an exercise mat is essential for comfortable and safe isometric training. Mats provide cushioning and support during floor exercises, making them more enjoyable and reducing the risk of injury.

Benefits:

- **Comfort:** Mats provide cushioning for your joints during exercises like planks, bridges, and seated holds, allowing for longer and more effective workouts.
- **Stability:** A non-slip surface ensures that you can maintain your grip and balance while performing isometric holds, reducing the likelihood of injury.
- **Versatile Use:** Mats can be used for a variety of exercises beyond isometric training, making them a valuable addition to any fitness routine.

When it comes to incorporating isometric exercise into your routine for managing high blood pressure, understanding the appropriate frequency and duration of workouts is crucial for achieving optimal results. Establishing a consistent practice can enhance the benefits of isometric training, support muscle development, and contribute to improved cardiovascular health.

Frequency of Isometric Workouts

For individuals aiming to lower blood pressure and strengthen muscles through isometric exercise, aiming for consistency is key. The general recommendation for most fitness programs is to engage in strength training exercises, including isometric workouts, at least **two to three times per week**. This frequency allows your muscles sufficient time to recover while still providing the necessary stimulus for growth and endurance.

However, for those specifically looking to manage high blood pressure, it's essential to consider personal factors such as current fitness levels, any underlying health conditions, and individual responses to exercise. Starting with **two sessions per week** can be an excellent foundation, gradually increasing to three or more as your strength and comfort levels improve.

It's also worth noting that some individuals may find success by integrating shorter isometric sessions into their daily routines. Performing isometric exercises every day, even for just 5-10 minutes, can provide cumulative benefits without overwhelming the body. For example, incorporating a few sets of wall sits or plank holds during breaks at work can help build strength and promote better blood flow throughout the day.

Duration of Isometric Workouts

The duration of each isometric exercise session is equally important. Research suggests that holding each isometric contraction for **15 to 30 seconds** is effective for most individuals, particularly those looking to improve strength and lower blood pressure. This time frame allows muscles to engage sufficiently to stimulate growth while keeping the intensity manageable.

Beginners may start with shorter holds, around **10-15 seconds**, focusing on maintaining proper form and technique. As strength and endurance increase, gradually extend the hold time to 30 seconds or longer. It's crucial to listen to your body—if you experience discomfort or fatigue, it's best to rest or reduce the duration.

For a comprehensive workout session, consider performing **2 to 4 sets** of each isometric exercise. Rest for about **30 to 60 seconds** between sets to allow your muscles to recover adequately. During this time, focus on controlled breathing to promote relaxation and maintain a steady heart rate, which is especially important for individuals managing high blood pressure.

Example Workout Structure

To help illustrate a structured approach to frequency and duration, consider the following example of a beginner isometric workout tailored for managing high blood pressure:

Frequency: 2-3 times per week

Duration: 20-30 minutes per session

CHAPTER 5

Types of Isometric Exercises for High Blood Pressure

Upper Body Exercises

Wall push-ups

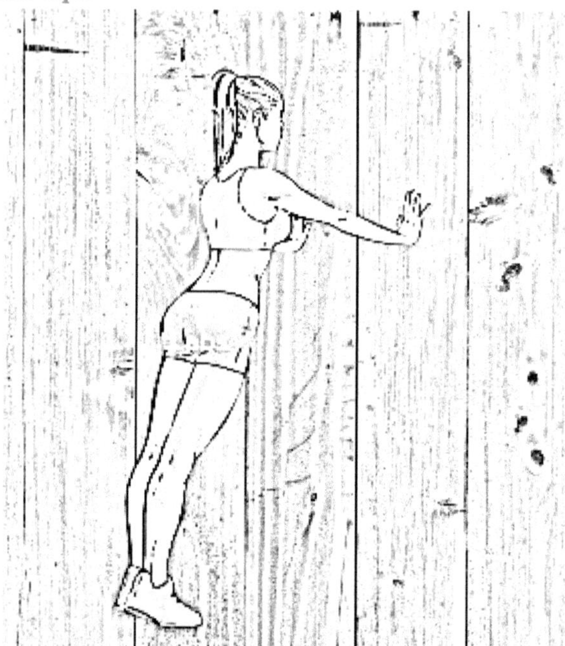

A straightforward but efficient isometric exercise that can help control high blood pressure is the wall push-up. This workout helps strengthen your upper body muscles without requiring a lot of activity, which can also help your cardiovascular system.

How to Complete Wall Push-Ups

- **Find a wall**: Find a wall that is around the height of your chest.
- **Choose a starting point:** Place your feet shoulder-width apart and face the wall. With your fingers pointing down, place your hands flat against the wall at shoulder height.
- **Bend forward**: Maintaining a straight posture and firmly planted feet, slowly bend forward. Keep bending until your chest almost touches the wall.
- **Hold your position**: For ten to fifteen seconds, or longer if your strength allows, maintain this posture.
- **Go back to where you were before**: Return to the starting position gradually while keeping your movement under control.
- **Repeat**: Depending on your level of fitness, perform this exercise ten to fifteen times or more.

Frequency

Wall push-ups should be done two to three times a week as part of your general workout regimen. In order to reap the rewards of this workout, consistency is essential.

Benefits of Wall push-ups

- Improves muscles of the upper body: Push-ups against a wall work your triceps, shoulders, and chest.
- Enhances cardiovascular health: Exerting yourself physically can help control blood pressure and strengthen your heart.
- Low impact: People with joint problems can benefit from this workout because it is mild on the joints.
- Simple to understand: People of all fitness levels can execute wall push-ups, which are an easy activity.

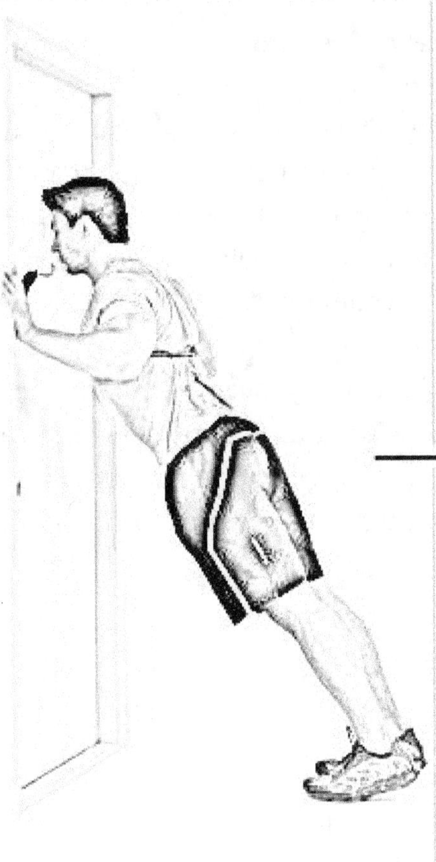

One kind of isometric exercise that can help control high blood pressure is the doorway push-up. By tightening your muscles without using them, isometric exercises help build muscle strength and endurance without raising your heart rate excessively.

How to Complete Doorway push-ups

- **Locate a doorway**. Select a doorway that has a strong doorframe.
- Put your hands shoulder-height on the doorframe with your palms flat against the frame.
- **Move forward**: Take a step forward until your body forms a straight line from your head to your feet and your arms are completely extended.
- **Bend forward**: Bend forward to the point when your chest nearly meets the doorframe.
- **Hold:** Maintain this posture for ten to fifteen seconds, or however long is comfortable for you.
- **Rest:** After a little break, repeat for a few times.

Frequency

Aim for two to three sets of ten to fifteen doorway push-ups, two to three times a week. As you gain strength, you can progressively increase the length of time or the quantity of sets.

Benefits of Doorway push-ups

- Enhances strength in the upper body: Doorway push-ups work the shoulders, triceps, and chest.
- Muscle endurance is increased: Maintaining the isometric contraction promotes endurance.
- Regularly performing isometric exercise has the potential to reduce blood pressure.
- Minimal equipment is needed: All you need for this exercise is a doorway.
- can to be completed anywhere: You can do doorway push-ups in your house, office, or any other place that has a doorway.

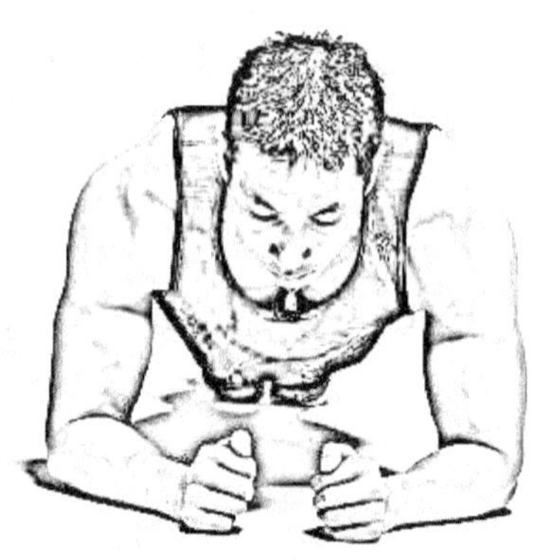

An isometric exercise called a plank calls on you to maintain a static posture while using your legs, glutes, and core. It's a powerful technique to enhance stability and balance, straighten your posture, and strengthen your core.

How to Complete Plank

- Put your hands directly beneath your shoulders with your fingers pointed forward to perform a push-up.
- Raising yourself off the ground: Involve your legs, glutes, and core as you push up onto your hands.
- Form a straight line: Keep your hips from rising or sagging by drawing a straight line from your head to your heels.
- Hold your position: Keep your body tight and your core active while you hold this position for as long as you can.

Frequency

Weekly goal: two to three plank practices, each lasting 15 to 30 seconds. Increase the duration gradually as your strength allows.

Benefits of Plank

- Strengthens core muscles: The transverse abdominis, obliques, and abdominals are among the many core muscles targeted by the plank.
- Proper posture can be improved and back discomfort can be decreased by performing planks on a regular basis.
- Increasing stability and balance is important because maintaining the plank position calls for a great deal of both.
- Helps control hypertension: By strengthening the musculature and enhancing general cardiovascular health, isometric exercises, such as planks, can help reduce hypertension.

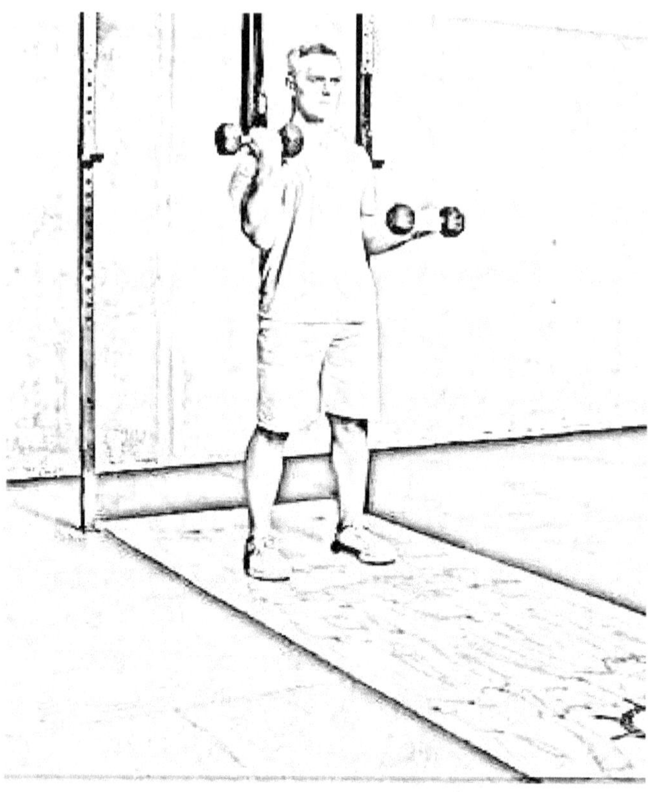

One kind of strength training exercise that includes contracting your biceps muscles without moving them is called an isometric bicep curl. This indicates that you are not moving dynamically; rather, you are maintaining a stationary position.

How to Complete Isometric bicep curls

- Place your arms by your sides as you stand: Maintain your palms pointing front and your feet shoulder-width apart.
- Bend your elbows: As you raise your forearms toward your shoulders, contract your biceps as though you were curling a weight.
- Hold your position: For ten to fifteen seconds, maintain an isometric contraction while holding your elbows at a 90-degree angle.
- Lower your arms slowly: Replicate from the beginning position.

Frequency

Try to get in two or three isometric bicep curl exercises a week, with ten to fifteen repetitions per set.

Benefits of Isometric bicep curls

- Strengthening of Biceps: By working the biceps muscles, this exercise helps build upper body strength.
- Strengthens grip: Doing isometric bicep curls can help you have a stronger grasp, which is useful for a variety of everyday tasks.
- Aids in the management of high blood pressure: By strengthening the muscles and enhancing general cardiovascular health, isometric workouts, such as bicep curls, can help lower blood pressure.

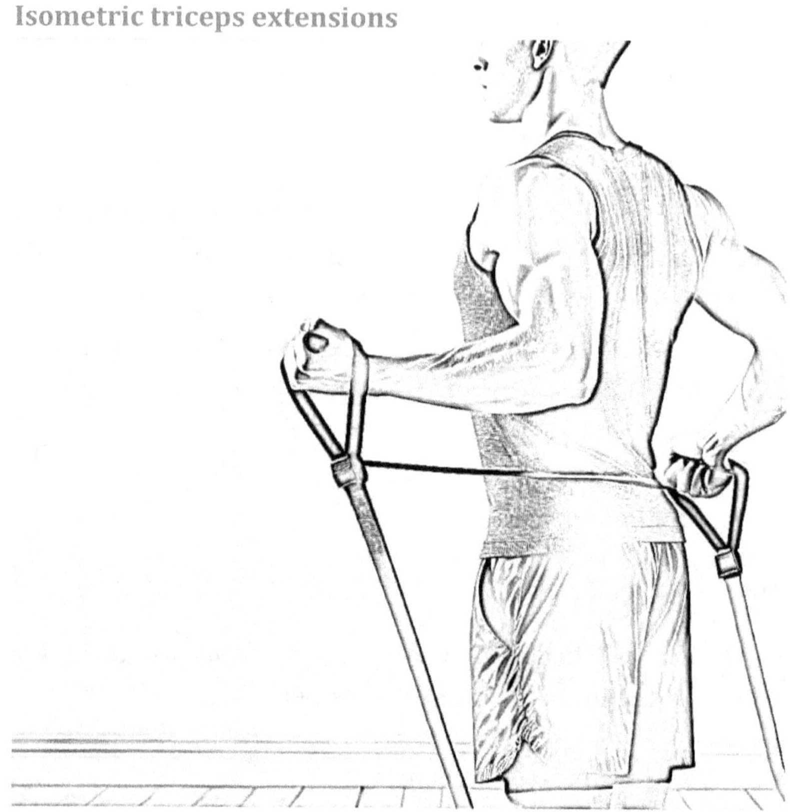

A straightforward but efficient workout that tones the triceps without needing a lot of movement is isometric triceps extensions. Because it improves muscle tone while preserving steady, controlled postures, this is especially advantageous for people who are controlling high blood pressure. Isometric exercises are a safe choice for people with cardiovascular difficulties because they don't need dynamic contractions, which may be done with little stress on the heart.

How to Complete Isometric Tricep Extensions

- Place your feet shoulder-width apart and stand straight with your back straight.
- Position a resistance band behind your back. Hold one end over your left shoulder and the other in your right hand, close to the base of your lower back.
- Using your left hand, pull the band upward while bending your elbow to a 90-degree angle. While your right hand is keeping the band firmly in place close to your lower back, your left hand should be tugging against the band's tension.
- Hold this position while keeping the band taut to activate your triceps muscles without moving.
- Maintain the posture for 15 to 30 seconds, making sure your core remains firm and your elbows close to your body.
- Change arms and carry out the motion again on the opposite side.
- Make sure to maintain perfect form throughout the workout as you perform 2-4 sets on each side.

Frequency

It is advised that those with high blood pressure execute isometric triceps extensions two to three times a week. This is an exercise that you can use alone or as part of an upper body fitness regimen. To give your muscles time to heal, make sure you take at least one day off in between workouts.

Benefits of Isometric Tricep Extensions

- Tightens the triceps: By focusing on the triceps muscles, isometric triceps extensions boost upper body strength.
- Enhances the endurance of muscles: Maintaining still postures increases triceps endurance.
- Encourages blood circulation: Although the workout does not require repetitive motion, it does aid in blood circulation stimulation, which is advantageous for controlling blood pressure.
- Low impact: This exercise is a good choice for people with high blood pressure because it puts less stress on the heart and joints.
- Practical and adaptable: This is a minimal equipment and space exercise that you can do at home, at the gym, or even at work.

Equipment Needed

All that is needed is a resistance band. Bands vary in resistance, so pick one that offers just the right amount of tension without being too tight.

Space Required

A tiny space that allows you to stand and spread your arms is what you'll need. Generally, three feet by three feet is a sufficient amount of room.

Assistance Required

Although novices may benefit from a trainer's supervision to ensure perfect form and technique, this exercise is typically performed alone. For people who have trouble moving their arms or shoulders, adjustments or help can be required.

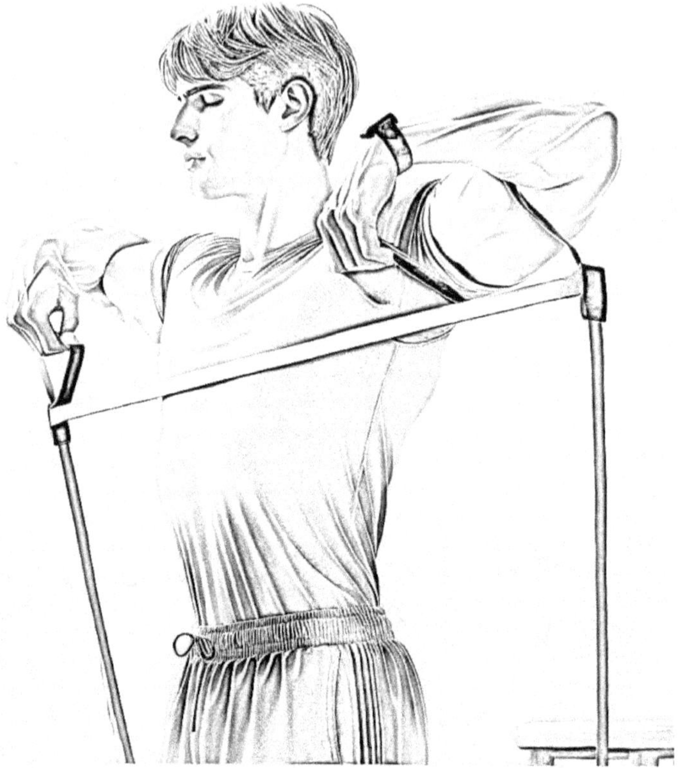

A static strength exercise that works the shoulders without requiring movement is the isometric shoulder press. This isometric variation differs from conventional pressing workouts in that it requires maintaining a posture that works the shoulder muscles. Because it strengthens the upper body and puts less burden on the heart than dynamic motions, it's a great workout for people with high blood pressure. The isometric shoulder press can enhance muscle endurance and stability by emphasizing regulated, sustained stress, both of which are advantageous for cardiovascular health in general.

How to Do Isometric shoulder press

- Start Position: Place your feet shoulder-width apart and stand erect. With your elbows 90 degrees bent and your palms facing forward, raise your arms to shoulder height.
- Engage Your Muscles: While maintaining the stance without moving your arms, push upwards as though you were pressing a heavy object overhead. The arms and shoulders should feel the strain.
- Maintain the Role: Hold the push for ten to thirty seconds while using your shoulder muscles.
- Rest and Release: Return to the starting position slowly, take a 30- to 60-second break, and then repeat.
- Repeat: Do two to four sets.

Frequency

Do the isometric shoulder press two to three times a week to properly control excessive blood pressure. Because shoulder muscles require time to recuperate, make sure you get enough rest in between exercises. Increase the hold's duration steadily over time.

Benefits of Isometric shoulder press

- Strengthens Shoulders: By keeping the muscles taut, this exercise increases shoulder strength and stability.
- Reduces Blood Pressure: It has been demonstrated that isometric workouts, such as the shoulder press, can help lower both the diastolic and systolic blood pressure.
- Boosts Endurance: Supports overall upper body performance by increasing shoulder muscular endurance.

Equipment Needed

There is no need for machines or weights. This exercise can be done using body weight, but a resistance band or light dumbbells can be used for added challenge.

Space Required

Just enough room is needed to completely stretch your arms without encountering any obstacles.

Assistance Required

No assistance is typically needed, making this exercise ideal for individuals to do at home or on their own.

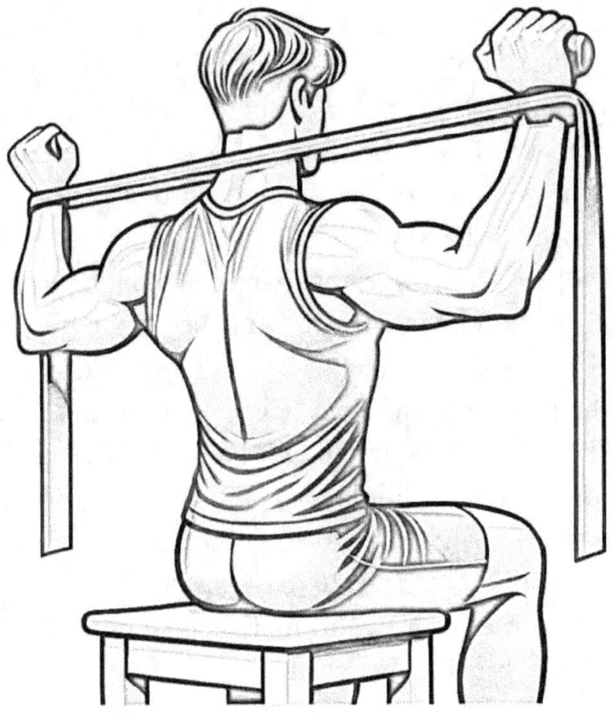

An efficient workout for the latissimus dorsi, or "lats," the big muscles in your back, is the isometric lat pulldown. In contrast to conventional lat pulldowns, this isometric variation entails holding the contraction motionless while drawing down against resistance. This static hold is perfect for enhancing posture and upper body strength because it strengthens and stabilizes the arms and back. Because isometric lat pulldowns concentrate on muscle tension rather than dynamic action, they improve the cardiovascular system without putting undue burden on the heart in people with high blood pressure.

How to Do Isometric lat pulldowns

- Starting Position: Place your feet level on the floor and sit with your back straight on a chair or bench.
- Grip the Resistance: Hold the center part above your head with both hands or secure it above you (for example, over a door or strong beam) with a resistance band.
- Pull Down: Lower both hands as though performing a standard lat pulldown, but pause in the middle.
- Hold the Position: For 15 to 30 seconds, maintain the pulling position by using your lat muscles. You should have your elbows pointed down and your arms bent at a 90-degree angle.
- Release: Return to the initial position after gradually releasing the tension.
- Again: Perform two to four sets, taking a 30- to 60-second break in between.

Frequency

It is advised to execute isometric lat pulldowns two to three times a week in order to manage high blood pressure. With an emphasis on executing 2-4 sets and holding each contraction for 15-30 seconds, each exercise should last roughly 15 to 20 minutes.

Benefits of Isometric lat pulldowns

- Enhances Upper Body Strength: It efficiently targets the latissimus dorsi, strengthening the back muscles.
- Enhances Posture: This exercise helps to improve posture by using the back muscles.
- Promotes Cardiovascular Health: By strengthening muscles without unduly increasing heart rate, it can help lower blood pressure, just like other isometric workouts.
- Low Impact: This exercise is perfect for persons with hypertension who need to avoid high-impact activities because it is easy on the joints.

Equipment Needed

- A cable machine or resistance band.
- If employing a resistance band, a strong anchor point.

Space Required

You only need enough area to sit or stand with your arms outstretched overhead for this workout. A tiny space in the living room or home gym might be adequate.

Assistance Required

This is an easy activity that you can complete on your own. Beginners, however, might benefit from assistance in fastening the resistance band or ensuring correct form.

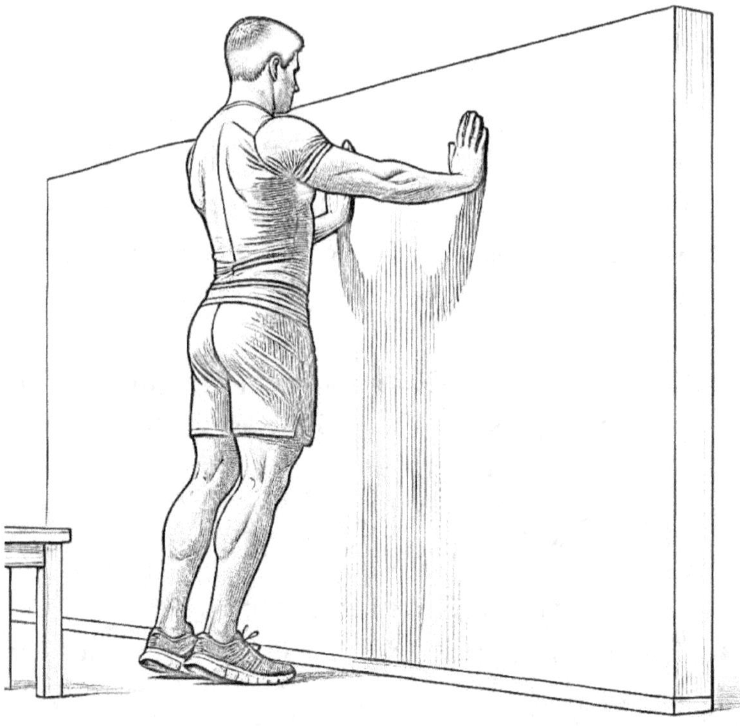

An efficient exercise that works the chest muscles without requiring dynamic movement is the isometric chest press. If you want to control your high blood pressure and increase your power, it might be a useful addition to your routine. A safe and regulated method of working the upper body, the chest press supports cardiovascular health in general.

How to Do Isometric chest press

Position yourself

- Place your feet shoulder-width apart and face a solid wall.
- With your elbows bent at a 90-degree angle, place your palms flat against the wall at chest height.
- To stay stable, make sure your back is straight and use your core.

Engage Your Muscles

- As if you were trying to push the wall away, press your palms against it.
- Without moving your body, concentrate on tensing your arm, shoulder, and chest muscles.
- Make sure you're not leaning on the wall and maintain the same elbow angle.

Hold the position

- For 15 to 30 seconds, continue pressing while maintaining tension in your upper body muscles.
- To prevent holding your breath, which might result in blood pressure increases, keep in mind to breathe steadily during the hold.

Release the Pressure

- After the hold, relax your arms and chest to gradually relieve the strain.
- Before beginning the following set, take a 30- to 60-second break and shake up your arms if necessary.

Repeat

Depending on your comfort level and degree of fitness, complete two to four sets of the exercise.

Frequency

It is advised that people with high blood pressure incorporate the isometric chest press into their exercise regimen two to three times per week. Two to four sets of presses, each held for 15 to 30 seconds, should make up each session. As your strength increases, gradually lengthen each hold.

Benefits of Isometric chest press

- Enhances Muscle Strength: By strengthening your pectoral muscles, shoulders, and triceps, the chest press helps you develop better posture and strength in your upper body.
- Promotes Cardiovascular Health: By increasing muscular tone and blood circulation, frequent isometric exercise can lower blood pressure.
- Low Impact on Joints: This exercise is ideal for people with joint pain or restricted mobility because it doesn't involve any movement, which makes it easy on the joints.
- Enhances Core Stability: By maintaining appropriate form, the chest press also engages your core muscles, helping to overall stability.

Equipment Needed

All you need is a strong wall. Because no special equipment is required, anyone, anywhere, can perform this workout.

Space Required

You just need enough room in front of a wall to stretch your arms and stay balanced. A living room, office, or any other space with a wall can be used for this.

Assistance Required

An easy exercise that doesn't require any help is the isometric chest press. To guarantee correct technique, novices can benefit from having a partner or teacher offer feedback on their form.

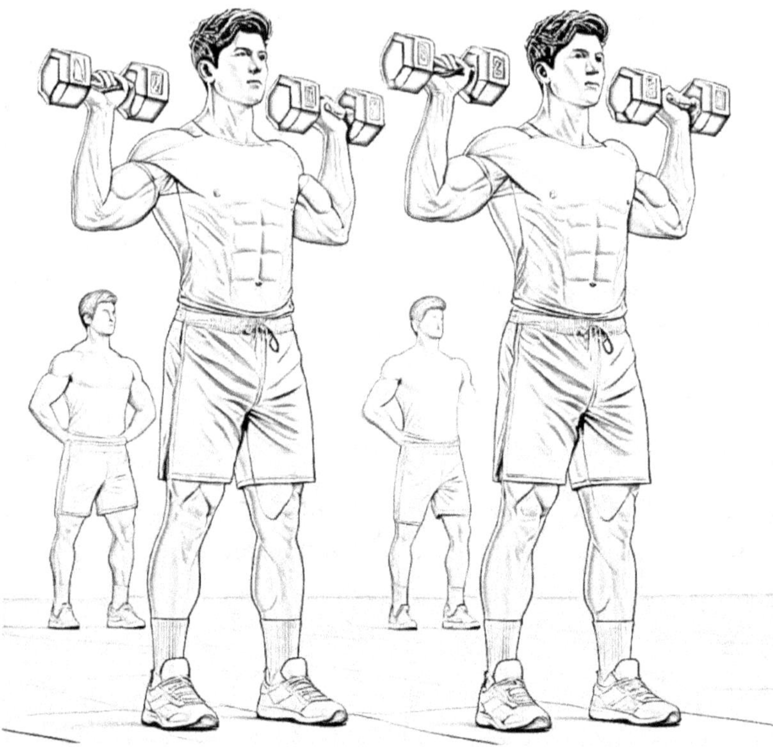

Through static muscle contraction, the isometric overhead press helps lower blood pressure while strengthening the shoulders, upper chest, and triceps. In order to create muscle tension without causing joint movement, it entails holding weights or resistance bands motionless.

How to Do Isometric overhead press

- Start Position: Hold dumbbells or resistance bands at shoulder height while standing with your feet shoulder-width apart. Depending on comfort, you should have your elbows bent and your hands facing either front or inward.
- Engage Core: To stabilize your torso, maintain a tight core and contract your abdominal muscles.
- Press Upward: Before your arms are fully extended, stop pushing the weights or bands upward. Maintain a small 90-degree bend in your elbows to release tension in your shoulder muscles.
- Hold Position: Depending on your stamina and strength, hold this overhead posture for 15 to 30 seconds. Throughout the hold, concentrate on breathing deliberately.
- Lower and Rest: Return the weights to shoulder height gradually, take a 30- to 60-second break, and then repeat for two to four sets.

Frequency

To guarantee muscle recovery, perform the isometric overhead press two to three times a week, with at least one day off in between. As strength increases, beginners should gradually go to 4 sets of 15-second holds and hold for 30 seconds.

Benefits of Isometric overhead press

- Increased Shoulder Strength: Enhances the stability and functionality of the upper body by strengthening the deltoid muscles.
- Blood Pressure Control: By enhancing circulation and vascular health, static holds in isometric workouts assist lower blood pressure.
- Improved Muscle Endurance: Maintaining the posture helps with posture and general strength by increasing upper body endurance.
- Core Stability: By strengthening the lower back and abdominal muscles during the activity, the core improves body control.

Equipment Needed

The most popular equipment for this workout is resistance bands or dumbbells (low to medium weight).

As an alternative, you can use any household object that has some weight, like water bottles.

Space Required

A compact area of around 4 by 4 feet is adequate. You must have sufficient space to stand and raise your arms above your head without any hindrance.

Assistance Required

Having a knowledgeable partner or a teacher can help novices avoid tension and maintain perfect form. But after you're comfortable with the method, you can work on this practice by yourself.

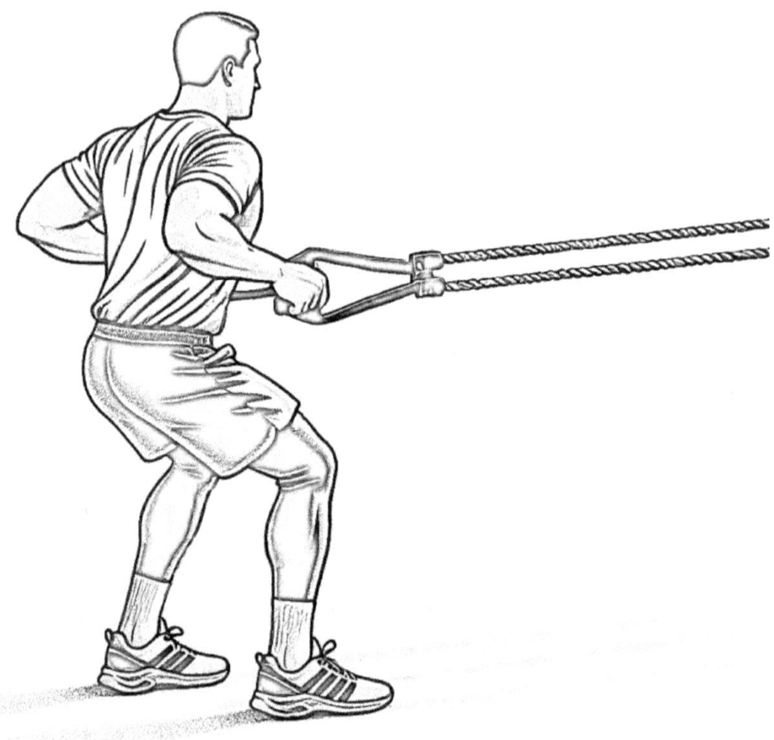

An excellent option for increasing strength without requiring a lot of activity is the isometric row, which targets the arms, shoulders, and back muscles. Through the use of static holds, this low-impact exercise can help people with high blood pressure maintain their cardiovascular health and muscle endurance without placing an unnecessary burden on their hearts.

How to Do Isometric Row

Starting Position

- To ensure a sturdy platform, place your feet shoulder-width apart.
- Grab a bar, resistance band, or other sturdy item that you can pull against.
- Maintain a straight back and slightly bend your knees while maintaining an active core.

Pulling Motion

- Bring the resistance band or object closer to your torso by bending your arms at the elbows.
- Maintain a 90-degree angle with your arms, keeping your elbows close to your sides.

Engage Your Muscles:

- Maintain the posture while concentrating on tightening your arms, shoulders, and back muscles.
- Throughout the hold, keep your posture straight, engage your core, and breathe steadily.

Hold the Position

- For 15 to 30 seconds, maintain the isometric contraction while concentrating on regulated breathing and taut muscles.

Release

- Return to the initial position after gradually releasing the tension.

Frequency

The isometric row should be performed two to three times a week for people who are controlling high blood pressure. There can be two to four sets in a session, with each hold lasting fifteen to thirty seconds. Between sets, take a 30- to 60-second break to let your muscles rest.

Benefits of Isometric Row

- Strengthens Upper Body Muscles: Encourages improved posture and muscular balance by activating the arms, shoulders, and back.
- Promotes Cardiovascular Health: This exercise is appropriate for people with high blood pressure since it increases muscle

endurance without raising heart rate by concentrating on static holds.

- Enhances Core Stability: By activating the core, the isometric row also enhances general body stability.
- Low Impact: The workout is joint-friendly and lowers the chance of injury because it doesn't require dynamic movement.

Equipment Needed

- Resistance Band: Typically, a straightforward band is fastened to a sturdy object.
- Sturdy Bar or Object: Any strong object that provides resistance when pulled against can be used.

Space Required

The isometric row requires very little space. Make sure you have adequate space to stand and spread your arms wide.

Assistance Required

This activity usually doesn't require any help. To make sure they are using the right muscles, beginners could benefit from having someone walk them through good form at first.

Wall sit

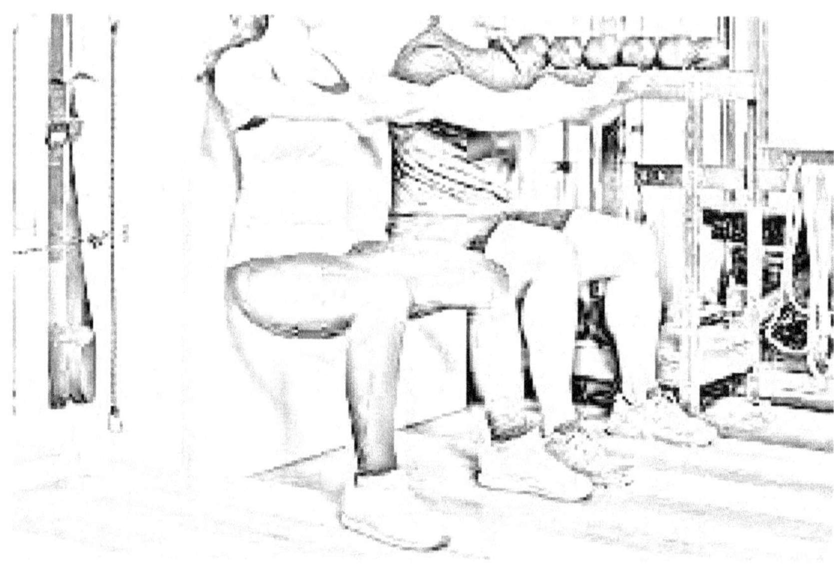

An efficient isometric exercise for controlling high blood pressure is the wall sit. Wall sits work the lower body muscles without creating abrupt increases in heart rate because the thighs are kept in a static position with the ground parallel to them. Isometric workouts have been shown to enhance vascular function, which eventually lowers resting blood pressure. This kind of exercise improves circulation and strengthens the muscles, which lessens the strain on the heart. It's an easy, low-impact choice for people who want to increase their muscle endurance and control their blood pressure.

How to Do Wall sit

- Locate a Wall: Position yourself against a solid wall with your back flat.
- Position Yourself: Your thighs should be parallel to the floor as you slide down the wall. A 90-degree bend should be made in your knees.
- Engage Core: Make sure your back stays flat on the wall and maintain a tight core.
- Hold the Position: Depending on your strength level, hold this position for as long as you can, aiming for 20 to 60 seconds.
- Get Up Slowly: Push yourself away from the wall as you slowly get back up.

Frequency

- Novices: two to three times per week, maintaining the posture for 20 to 30 seconds.
- Advanced: Holding the pose for more than 60 seconds up to four or five times per week.

Benefits of wall sits

- Lower Blood Pressure: By enhancing vascular health, isometric workouts such as wall sits can help lower high blood pressure.
- Strengthens Lower Body: Focuses on the glutes, hamstrings, and quadriceps.
- Enhances Endurance: Increases muscle endurance, which can lead to improved physical performance in day-to-day tasks.

- Minimal Impact on Joints: This exercise is appropriate for people with joint problems because it is static and puts less strain on joints.

Equipment Needed

A solid, level wall.

Space Required

Just enough room to stretch your legs and lean against a wall.

Assistance Required

In most cases, no support is required, but novices might want someone to keep an eye on their form.

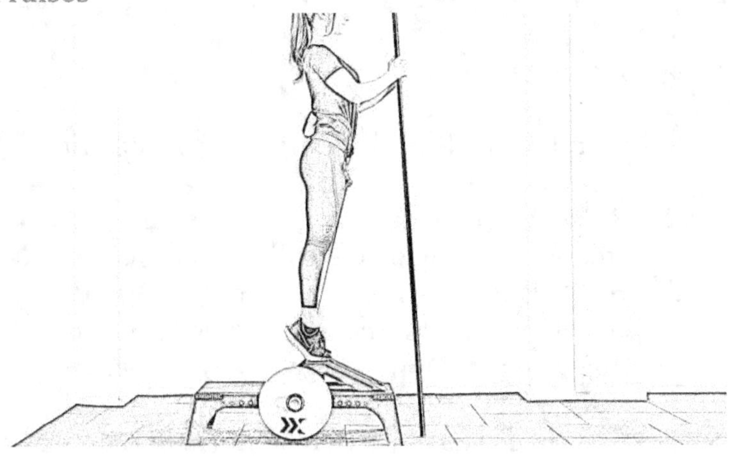

A straightforward yet powerful exercise for strengthening the lower leg muscles, especially the gastrocnemius and soleus, is the calf raise. They require using the calf muscles to keep balance and stability while standing on the balls of the feet and raising the heels off the ground. Calf raises are beneficial for everyday tasks as well as sports performance since they can increase circulation, ankle strength, and muscular tone. By encouraging improved blood flow and vascular health, they can also aid in the management of high blood pressure when done isometrically (keeping the body lifted).

Calf Raises as an Isometric Exercise for High Blood Pressure
Steps to Perform It:

1. **Stand Upright**: Position your feet hip-width apart and stand tall.
2. **Raise Your Heels**: Slowly lift your heels off the ground, standing on the balls of your feet.
3. **Hold**: Hold this raised position for 10-30 seconds, keeping your core engaged and body balanced.
4. **Lower Back Down**: Slowly lower your heels back to the ground.
5. **Repeat**: Perform 10-15 repetitions in each set.

Frequency:

- **Beginner**: 2-3 times a week with shorter hold times (10-15 seconds).
- **Advanced**: 4-5 times a week, holding for 30+ seconds.

Benefits:

- **Improves Circulation**: Isometric exercises like calf raises promote blood flow, which can help reduce high blood pressure.
- **Strengthens Calf Muscles**: Enhances muscle strength and endurance in the lower legs.
- **Joint-Friendly**: A low-impact movement that places minimal stress on the joints, making it suitable for various fitness levels.

Equipment Needed:

- None, but a chair or wall for balance is helpful.

Space Required:

- Only enough room to stand comfortably and lift your heels.

Assistance Required:

- None required, though beginners might benefit from light support, like touching a wall or chair for balance.

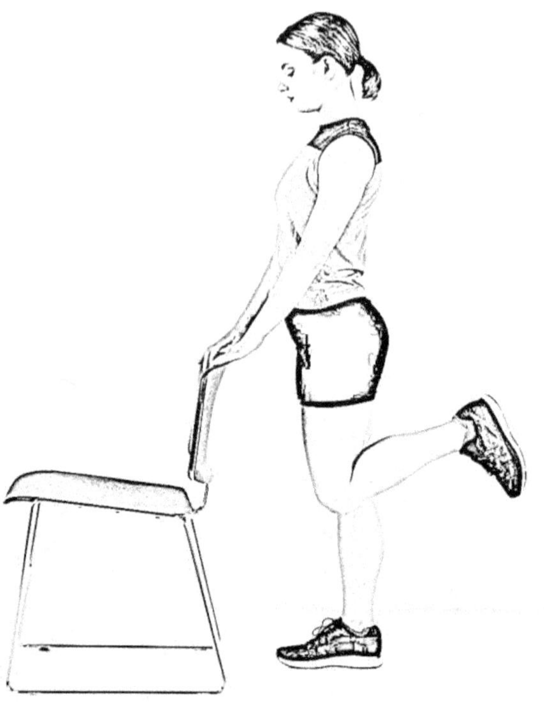

Hamstring curls are a simple but effective way to target the hamstring muscles. They can be performed in various forms, either with dynamic movements or as isometric holds. In isometric versions, holding the bent leg position engages the hamstrings, promoting strength and endurance while reducing the risk of injury.

Steps to Perform It:

1. **Stand Upright**: Find a sturdy surface, like a wall or chair, to hold onto for balance.
2. **Bend One Leg**: Lift one leg by bending at the knee, bringing your heel toward your glutes.
3. **Hold the Position**: Hold the position where you feel your hamstring muscle is engaged. Your back must be kept straight and your core tight.
4. **Switch Legs**: After holding the position for 20-30 seconds, slowly lower your leg and switch to the other side.

Frequency:

- **Beginners**: 2-3 times a week, holding each leg for 20-30 seconds.
- **Advanced**: 4-5 times a week, holding for 45-60 seconds per leg.

Benefits:

- **Lower Blood Pressure**: Isometric hamstring curls help in lowering blood pressure by improving vascular function.
- **Strengthens Hamstrings**: Improves the strength and endurance of the hamstrings without high-impact movements.
- **Joint-Friendly**: It's low-impact, so it doesn't place stress on the knees or other joints.
- **Balance Improvement**: Holding the position helps enhance balance and stability.

Equipment Needed:

- None, though a wall or chair can be used for support.

Space Required:

- Just enough room to stand and bend your leg.

Assistance Required:

- Generally, no assistance is needed, but beginners may use support for balance.

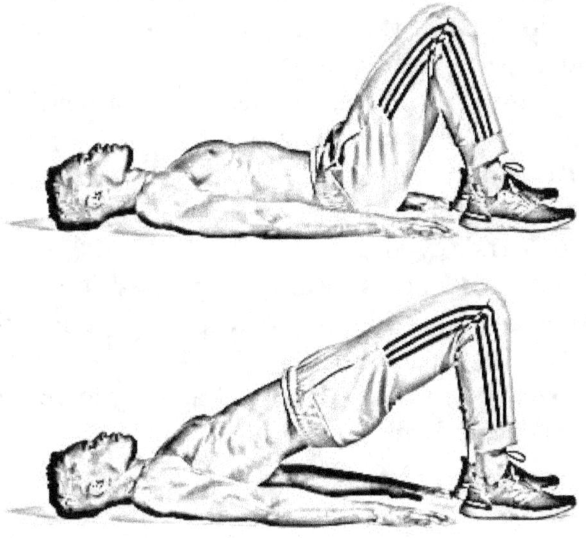

The glute bridge is a simple yet effective exercise that targets the gluteal muscles, core, and lower back. It involves lifting the hips off the ground while lying on your back, creating a bridge-like position. This exercise helps strengthen the posterior chain, improve posture, and enhance stability. As an isometric exercise, it's particularly beneficial for managing high blood pressure by improving circulation and cardiovascular health through static muscle engagement. The glute bridge is low-impact, making it suitable for people of all fitness levels.

Steps to Perform It:

1. Start by lying flat on your back with your feet flat on the floor, hip-width apart, and your knees bent.
2. **Position Your Arms**: Place your arms by your sides, palms facing down.
3. **Engage Your Core**: Tighten your core muscles and press your feet into the ground.
4. **Lift Your Hips**: Raise your hips toward the ceiling until your body forms a straight line from your shoulders to your knees.
5. **Hold the Position**: Maintain this position, squeezing your glutes and keeping your core tight for 20-60 seconds.
6. **Lower Your Hips Slowly**: Gradually lower your hips back down to the ground.

Frequency:

- **Beginners**: 2-3 times a week, holding the bridge for 20-30 seconds.
- **Advanced**: 4-5 times a week, holding for 60+ seconds.

Benefits:

- **Lower Blood Pressure**: Isometric holds can improve vascular health, helping to reduce high blood pressure.
- **Strengthens the Core and Glutes**: Targets the glute muscles, lower back, and core, enhancing strength and stability.
- **Improves Posture**: By strengthening the posterior chain, it helps improve posture and relieve lower back pain.

- **Low Impact**: Safe for individuals with joint concerns, as there's no impact on the knees or hips.

Equipment Needed:

- No equipment is needed, though a yoga mat can make the exercise more comfortable.

Space Required:

- Only enough space to lie down on your back comfortably.

Assistance Required:

- No assistance is generally required, but beginners may want to check their form with a mirror or trainer.

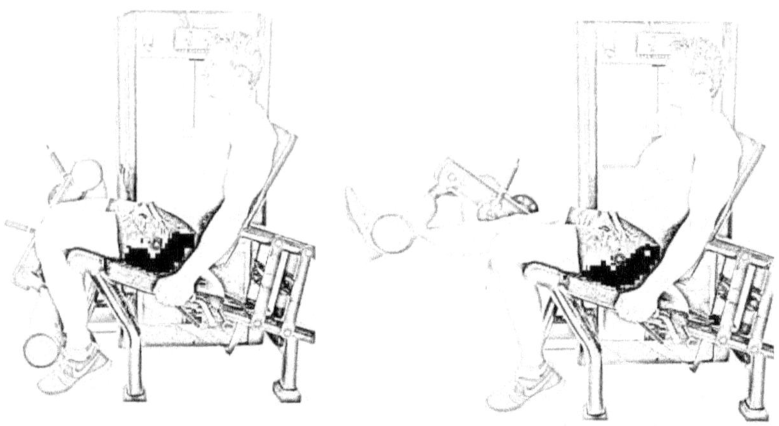

This exercise focuses on statically engaging the quadriceps while seated, helping build muscle strength and endurance. It is particularly beneficial for improving blood flow and can help reduce blood pressure with regular practice. The simplicity of the movement makes it accessible for most fitness levels.

Steps to Perform It:

1. **Seated Position**: Sit on a sturdy chair with your back straight and feet flat on the ground.
2. **Lift One Leg**: Extend one leg forward until it is straight and parallel to the floor, keeping the foot flexed.
3. **Hold**: Tighten your thigh muscles and hold the position for 10-30 seconds.
4. **Switch Legs**: Lower the leg back to the ground and repeat with the opposite leg.
5. **Repeat**: Alternate between legs for the desired number of repetitions.

Frequency:

- **Beginners**: 2-3 times per week, 3 sets of 10-20 seconds per leg.
- **Advanced**: 4-5 times per week, 3 sets of 30+ seconds per leg.

Benefits:

- **Lower Blood Pressure**: Holding static positions helps improve circulation and reduce blood pressure over time.
- **Strengthens Quadriceps**: Targets the quadriceps, making it effective for strengthening the front of the thigh.
- **Joint-Friendly**: Since it's a static movement, it is gentle on the knee joints, making it suitable for those with joint concerns.

Equipment Needed:

- A sturdy chair.

Space Required:

- Small space, just enough for a chair and leg extension.

Assistance Required:

- Generally no assistance required, but beginners may want support with balance initially.

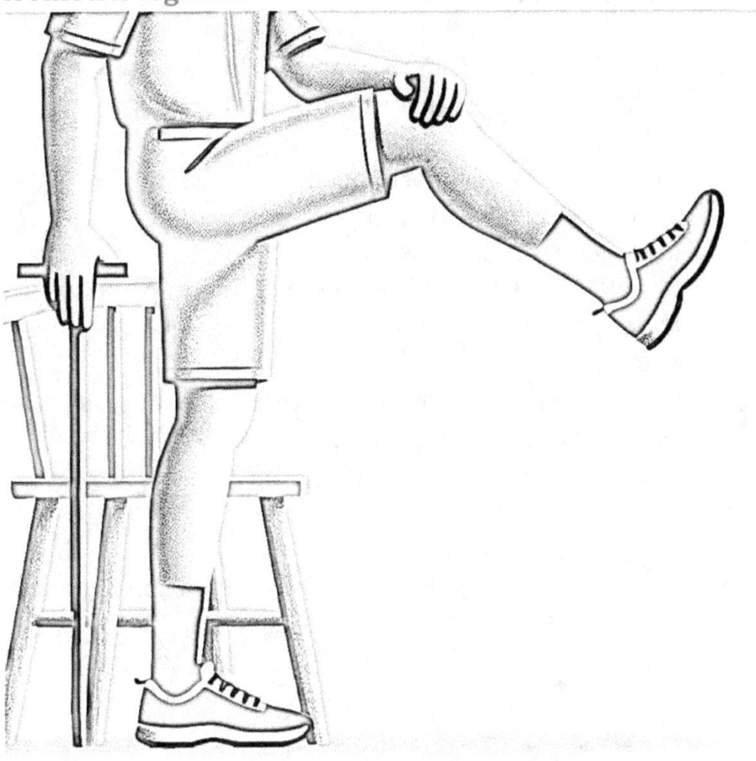

Isometric leg curls focus on strengthening the hamstring muscles through static contraction. Holding the bent position works the muscles without actual movement, which can be useful for those with joint concerns. By adding regular isometric leg curls to a fitness routine, individuals can improve muscle tone and endurance while supporting better blood pressure control.

Steps to Perform It:

1. **Start Position**: Stand straight with feet shoulder-width apart, using a sturdy object (like a chair) for balance.
2. **Bend One Leg**: Slowly bend one leg at the knee, bringing the heel toward your buttocks. Keep the other leg straight for support.
3. **Hold the Position**: Keep the bent leg in position, feeling the tension in your hamstring. Maintain the hold for 20-30 seconds.
4. **Switch Legs**: Return the leg to the starting position and repeat on the other leg.

Frequency:

- **Beginners**: 2-3 times a week, holding each leg curl for 20-30 seconds.
- **Advanced**: Up to 4-5 times a week, holding each curl for 45-60 seconds.

Benefits:

- **Blood Pressure Management**: Isometric exercises can help reduce high blood pressure through sustained muscle tension, improving vascular health.
- **Hamstring Strength**: Targets and strengthens the hamstring muscles without any dynamic movement.
- **Improved Stability**: Enhances balance and stability, particularly important for those with weak or stiff muscles.
- **Low Impact**: Gentle on the joints and suitable for people with joint or mobility issues.

Equipment Needed:

* A chair or other sturdy object for balance.

Space Required:

* A small area enough to stand and extend your leg.

Assistance Required:

* Generally, no assistance is needed, but beginners might benefit from someone watching for correct posture.

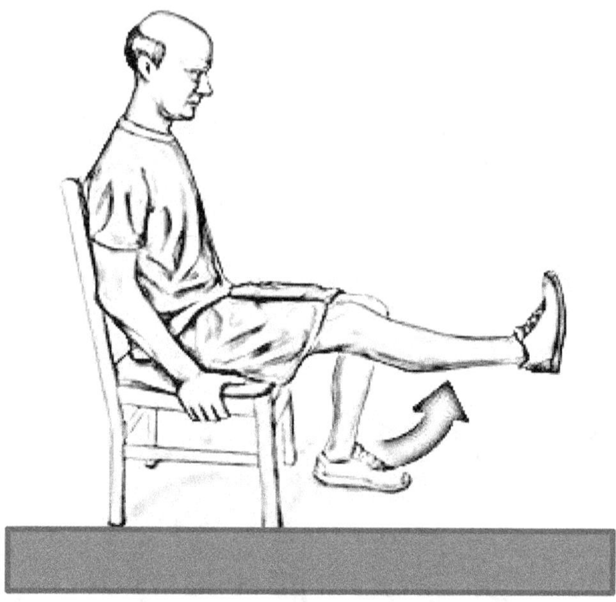

Isometric quadriceps contractions involve tensing the quadriceps without moving the knee joint. This form of exercise is particularly useful for individuals looking to strengthen their legs without putting strain on the knees. It's also effective in helping manage high blood pressure, as it promotes vascular health and improves blood flow while keeping the body in a stationary position.

Steps to Perform It:

1. **Sit or Lie Down**: Start by sitting on a chair or lying down on a flat surface with your legs extended.
2. **Engage Quadriceps**: Tighten or contract your quadriceps muscles (the muscles at the front of your thighs) without moving your leg. Focus on squeezing the muscle as hard as you can.
3. **Hold the Contraction**: Hold the contraction for 5-10 seconds.
4. **Release**: Slowly relax the muscle and rest for a few seconds.
5. **Repeat**: Perform the contraction 10-15 times per leg.

Frequency:

- **Beginners**: 2-3 sets per leg, 3 times a week.
- **Advanced**: 4-5 sets per leg, 4-5 times a week.

Benefits:

- **Blood Pressure Control**: Isometric exercises, like quadriceps contractions, can reduce high blood pressure by improving circulation and reducing the stress on the cardiovascular system.
- **Strengthens Quadriceps**: Focuses on strengthening the quadriceps muscles without joint movement, ideal for individuals with joint or mobility issues.
- **Improves Muscle Endurance**: Increases muscle endurance in the legs, which helps in daily activities such as walking or climbing stairs.

Equipment Needed:

- None, though a chair or a flat surface can be used for support.

Space Required:

- Minimal space, just enough to sit or lie down comfortably.

Assistance Required:

- Generally, no assistance is required, but beginners may benefit from supervision to ensure proper engagement of the quadriceps.

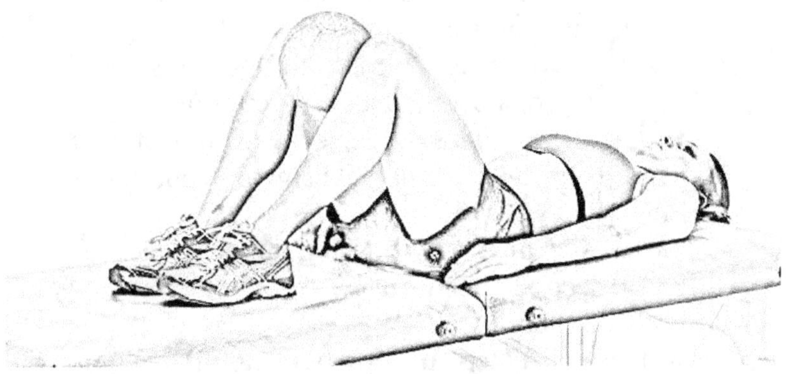

Isometric inner thigh contractions are a static exercise that focuses on strengthening the adductor muscles in the inner thighs without any movement. This exercise is beneficial for toning and stabilizing the lower body and has been found to aid in lowering high blood pressure, thanks to its positive effect on blood vessel flexibility and circulation. The simplicity and low impact of this exercise make it suitable for most fitness levels.

Steps to Perform It:

1. **Sit or Lie down Comfortably**: Find a chair or lie down with your feet hip-width apart.
2. **Position an Object**: Place a soft object, such as a pillow or yoga block, between your knees.
3. **Engage Inner Thighs**: Squeeze the object gently using your inner thighs, focusing on contracting the muscles.
4. **Hold the Contraction**: Maintain the squeeze for 15-30 seconds, focusing on keeping the rest of your body relaxed.
5. **Release and Repeat**: Slowly release the contraction, rest for a few seconds, and repeat the process.

Frequency:

- **Beginners**: Perform 2-3 sets, holding for 15-20 seconds each, 2-3 times a week.
- **Advanced**: Increase to 3-5 sets, holding for up to 30-60 seconds, 3-4 times a week.

Benefits:

- **Blood Pressure Reduction**: Regularly engaging in isometric exercises like inner thigh contractions can help lower blood pressure by improving circulation and relaxing blood vessels.
- **Strengthens Inner Thighs**: This exercise specifically targets and tones the adductor muscles of the inner thighs.
- **Low Impact**: Ideal for people with joint pain or mobility limitations, as it doesn't involve any movement or impact on the joints.

- **Improves Stability**: Strengthens muscles that contribute to balance and posture.

Equipment Needed:

- A soft object like a pillow, yoga block, or ball to squeeze between your legs.

Space Required:

- Minimal space is needed, enough for sitting or standing comfortably.

Assistance Required:

- Typically no assistance is required, making it an easy exercise to perform solo.

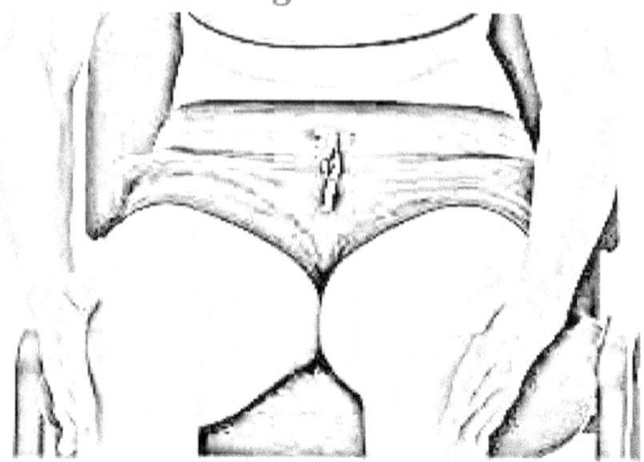

Isometric outer thigh contractions focus on activating the abductor muscles in the outer thighs. This exercise helps improve leg stability and strength while being gentle on the joints. It can be beneficial for individuals with high blood pressure, as static muscle contractions have been shown to improve heart health by reducing stress on the cardiovascular system.

Steps to Perform It:

1. **Seated Position**: Sit upright in a chair with your feet flat on the floor and legs slightly apart.
2. **Position Your Hands**: Place your hands on the outer sides of your thighs.
3. **Push Outward**: Press your thighs outward against the resistance of your hands without moving your legs. Hold the contraction.
4. **Engage the Muscles**: Focus on tightening the muscles in your outer thighs and hips.
5. **Hold and Release**: Hold this position for 10-30 seconds, then slowly release the tension and relax.

Frequency:

- **Beginners**: Perform 2-3 sets of 10-20 second holds, 3-4 times per week.
- **Advanced**: Increase to 4-5 sets of 30-second holds, 4-5 times per week.

Benefits:

- **Lower Blood Pressure**: Helps in reducing high blood pressure by enhancing circulation and vascular strength.
- **Strengthens Outer Thigh Muscles**: Targets the abductor muscles, improving leg stability and strength.
- **Joint-Friendly**: Low impact on the joints, making it ideal for those with joint issues or mobility concerns.
- **Improves Muscle Endurance**: Enhances the endurance of the outer thigh and hip muscles, aiding in better balance and stability.

Equipment Needed:

- No equipment required, but a sturdy chair is recommended.

Space Required:

- Minimal space needed, just enough to sit in a chair.

Assistance Required:

- No assistance is required for this exercise.

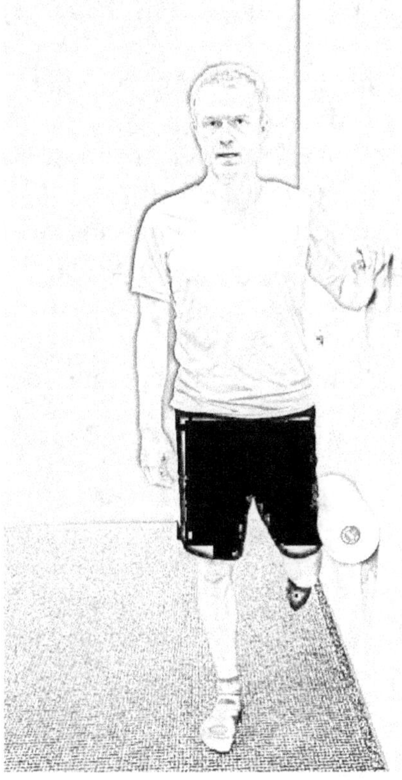

Isometric hip abductions involve holding the hip muscles in a contracted position without actual movement. This type of exercise strengthens the outer thighs and glutes while helping to stabilize the hips and improve balance. Regular practice can also contribute to better control over blood pressure.

1. **Start Position**: Stand upright with your feet hip-width apart, or lie on your side if doing a lying version.
2. **Engage the Core**: Tighten your core muscles to stabilize your body.
3. **Perform the Contraction**: Push your leg outward against resistance (such as a wall, resistance band, or immovable object) without moving it. Focus on contracting the outer thigh and hip muscles.
4. **Hold the Position**: Maintain this contraction for 10-30 seconds, keeping your core and hips engaged.
5. **Release**: Slowly relax the muscles and return to the starting position.
6. **Repeat**: Switch sides if needed and repeat the process.

Frequency:

- **Beginners**: 2-3 times a week, holding each contraction for 10-20 seconds.
- **Advanced**: 3-4 times a week, holding for 30+ seconds.

Benefits:

- **Improves Blood Pressure**: Isometric exercises have been shown to reduce blood pressure by improving circulation and reducing the heart's workload.
- **Strengthens Hip Muscles**: Targets hip abductors (outer thighs and glutes), improving stability and balance.
- **Joint-Friendly**: Because it's isometric, there's minimal joint movement, making it safe for those with joint concerns.

- **Postural Support**: Strengthens muscles that help with posture and daily activities.

Equipment Needed:

- None, or a resistance band for added tension.

Space Required:

- Minimal; enough space to stand or lie on the floor with some leg movement.

Assistance Required:

- No assistance is generally required, but supervision may be useful for beginners to ensure correct form.

Boat pose

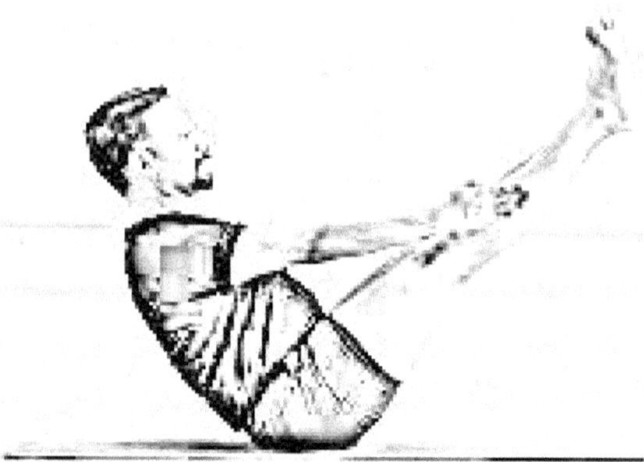

Boat pose, known as Navasana in yoga, is an excellent isometric exercise that focuses on building core strength. It involves balancing on your sitting bones while holding your legs and arms extended off the ground, creating a "V" shape with your body. The isometric contraction in this pose engages the deep core muscles, contributing to improved posture, stability, and circulation, which is especially helpful for individuals managing high blood pressure.

Steps to Perform It:

1. **Start seated:** Sit on the floor with your legs extended in front of you.
2. **Position your hands:** Place your hands on the floor beside your hips for support.
3. **Lift your legs:** Slowly lift your legs off the ground, keeping them straight or slightly bent, and bring them to about a 45-degree angle.
4. **Raise your arms:** Extend your arms parallel to the floor, reaching toward your feet, or keep them resting beside your hips if more stability is needed.
5. **Engage your core:** Tighten your abdominal muscles and maintain balance in this position.
6. **Hold the position:** Maintain this posture for 15-30 seconds, keeping your spine straight and your chest lifted.
7. **Relax:** After holding the position, slowly lower your legs and arms back to the starting position and rest for 30 seconds before repeating.

Frequency:

Boat pose contractions can be practiced **2-3 times per week** as part of your isometric exercise routine. Start by holding the position for 15 seconds, gradually increasing the time to 30 seconds or longer as you build core strength and endurance.

Benefits:

- **Improves cardiovascular health:** This pose strengthens core muscles, which indirectly supports blood circulation and helps regulate blood pressure.
- **Strengthens core muscles:** Boat pose effectively targets the abs, lower back, and hip flexors.

- **Enhances balance and stability:** Holding the pose improves overall stability and balance.
- **Reduces stress:** Focusing on the contraction during this pose promotes relaxation and reduces anxiety, which is beneficial for managing high blood pressure.

Equipment Needed:

- No equipment is needed to perform boat pose contractions, making it convenient to do anywhere.

Space Required:

- You only need enough floor space to fully extend your legs and arms, around 4-5 feet of clear space.

Assistance Required:

- No assistance is required, though beginners may benefit from using a yoga block or holding onto the back of their thighs for additional support.

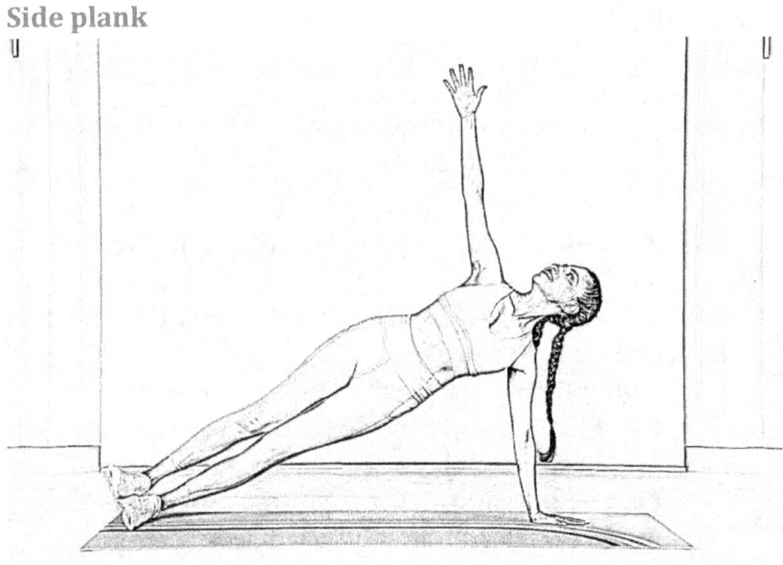

The side plank is a popular isometric exercise targeting the core muscles, particularly the obliques. This exercise helps improve balance and core strength, both of which are crucial for reducing the strain on the lower back and promoting better posture. Side planks can be especially beneficial for individuals with high blood pressure, as they provide a low-impact, strength-building activity that doesn't overly elevate the heart rate, allowing for safe and effective blood pressure management.

Steps to Perform It:

1. **Start on the floor:** Begin by lying on your side with your legs extended, one on top of the other. Place your elbow directly beneath your shoulder, with your forearm flat on the floor.
2. **Lift your hips:** Push your hips upward to form a straight line from your head to your feet. Only your forearm and the side of your bottom foot should be touching the ground.
3. **Engage your core:** Tighten your abdominal muscles to keep your body stable. Avoid letting your hips drop or sag.
4. **Hold the position:** Keep your body aligned and hold this position for 15-30 seconds or longer as you build strength.
5. **Lower your hips:** After completing the hold, slowly lower your hips back to the floor and switch to the other side for balance.

Frequency:

To support high blood pressure management, aim to perform side planks **2-3 times per week**. You can start with one set on each side, holding for 15-20 seconds, then gradually increase to 30 seconds or more as your core strength improves.

Benefits:

- **Lowers blood pressure:** Like other isometric exercises, side planks can help reduce resting blood pressure when practiced consistently.
- **Strengthens the core:** Side planks engage the obliques, lower back, and abdominal muscles, improving core stability.

- **Enhances posture:** Strengthening the core muscles helps maintain better posture and balance, reducing the strain on your back.
- **Increases endurance:** Holding the plank position for extended periods builds muscular endurance in the core and stabilizing muscles.

Equipment Needed:

- No equipment is necessary, although a yoga mat can be used for added comfort.

Space Required:

- You only need a small, flat area, about the length of your body, to perform side planks.

Assistance Required:

- Side planks are generally performed without assistance. Beginners may benefit from using a mirror or asking someone to check their form to ensure their body stays aligned.

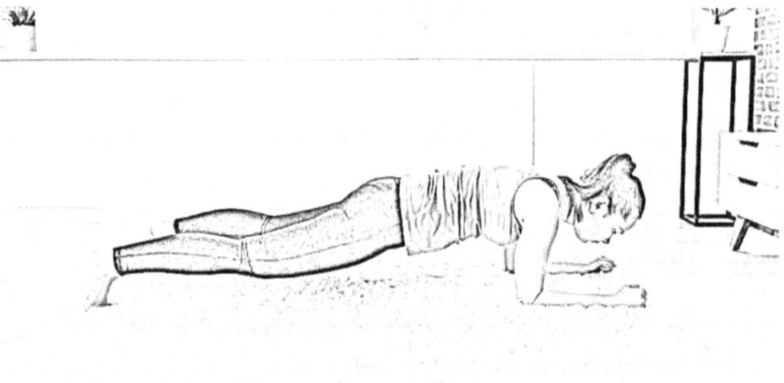

The isometric plank is a static exercise that strengthens multiple muscle groups without movement. It is particularly beneficial for those with high blood pressure because it engages large muscle groups in a way that improves circulation and reduces stress on the heart. As a full-body exercise, the plank strengthens the core, shoulders, arms, and legs while promoting better posture, which can aid in overall cardiovascular health

Steps to Perform It:

1. **Start on all fours:** Begin by kneeling on the floor with your hands placed directly under your shoulders.
2. **Position your feet:** Extend your legs straight behind you, balancing on your toes, with feet about hip-width apart.
3. **Align your body:** Keep your body in a straight line from your head to your heels, ensuring your hips don't sag or rise.
4. **Engage your core:** Tighten your abdominal muscles to maintain stability and prevent your back from arching.
5. **Hold the position:** Keep your forearms on the floor or hands flat, depending on the type of plank you're performing. Hold the position for 15-30 seconds.
6. **Breathe steadily:** While holding the plank, focus on maintaining steady, deep breaths.
7. **Release:** After holding the position for the desired time, lower yourself gently back to the floor.

Frequency:

To effectively manage high blood pressure, aim to include isometric planks in your workout **2-3 times per week**. Start with shorter hold times of 10-15 seconds and gradually increase to 30 seconds or more as your strength and endurance improve.

Benefits:

- **Lowers blood pressure:** Isometric planks, like other static exercises, can help reduce resting blood pressure.

- **Improves core strength:** The plank primarily engages the abdominal muscles, which enhances core stability.
- **Boosts endurance:** Holding the position for an extended time builds muscular endurance in the shoulders, arms, and core.
- **Increases posture and balance:** Planks promote proper posture by strengthening muscles along the spine.

Equipment Needed:

- No special equipment is required, though a **yoga mat** can provide comfort for your forearms and feet.

Space Required:

- The plank requires only minimal space, enough for your body to extend fully on the floor, approximately **6 feet by 3 feet**.

Assistance Required:

- No assistance is required to perform an isometric plank, though a timer or fitness app can help monitor your hold duration.

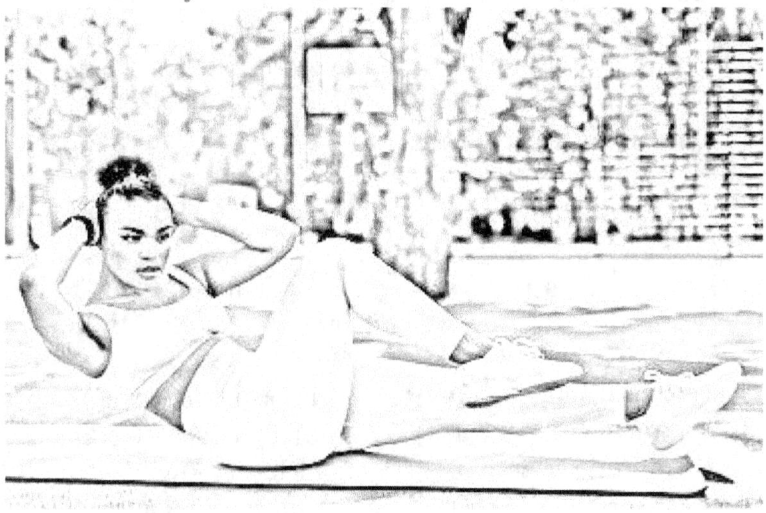

Isometric bicycle crunches focus on holding the contraction of the abdominal muscles while in a twisted position, rather than performing continuous movements. This variation helps build strength in the core while also promoting better blood circulation, making it an effective exercise for individuals seeking to manage high blood pressure through physical activity. The exercise emphasizes balance, core stability, and improved endurance, all without placing unnecessary strain on the cardiovascular system.

Steps to Perform It:

1. **Lie down:** Start by lying on your back on an exercise mat or a comfortable surface.
2. **Position your hands and legs:** Place your hands behind your head with your elbows out. Lift both legs off the ground, bending them at a 90-degree angle.
3. **Engage your core:** Tighten your abdominal muscles and lift your upper body slightly off the ground.
4. **Begin the movement:** Slowly bring your right knee toward your chest while simultaneously twisting your upper body to bring your left elbow toward your right knee. Hold the position without completing the full motion, keeping tension on the muscles.
5. **Hold the contraction:** Pause and hold the isometric contraction for **10 to 20 seconds** while keeping your core tight.
6. **Switch sides:** After holding the contraction, switch sides by bringing the left knee toward the right elbow. Hold this position again for 10-20 seconds.
7. **Return to starting position:** Lower your legs and upper body back to the mat, then repeat the process for the desired number of repetitions.

Frequency:

Isometric bicycle crunches can be performed **2-3 times per week** as part of your overall isometric exercise routine for managing high blood pressure. Start with 2-3 sets of 10-20 second holds on each side and increase as your endurance improves.

Benefits:

- **Improves cardiovascular health:** Engaging the core muscles through isometric holds can help enhance blood flow, indirectly supporting better blood pressure regulation.
- **Strengthens core muscles:** This exercise targets the abdominal muscles, helping improve core strength and stability.
- **Promotes balance and posture:** The twisting motion improves muscle coordination and balance, which is essential for overall physical health.
- **Low-impact:** Isometric bicycle crunches provide a core workout without causing unnecessary stress on the joints, making them suitable for individuals managing blood pressure.

Equipment Needed:

- An exercise mat or soft surface to lie on.

Space Required:

- A small space, about the size of a yoga mat, is sufficient for performing this exercise.

Assistance Required:

- This exercise typically requires no assistance. However, beginners might benefit from a timer to track hold times or a partner to ensure proper form.

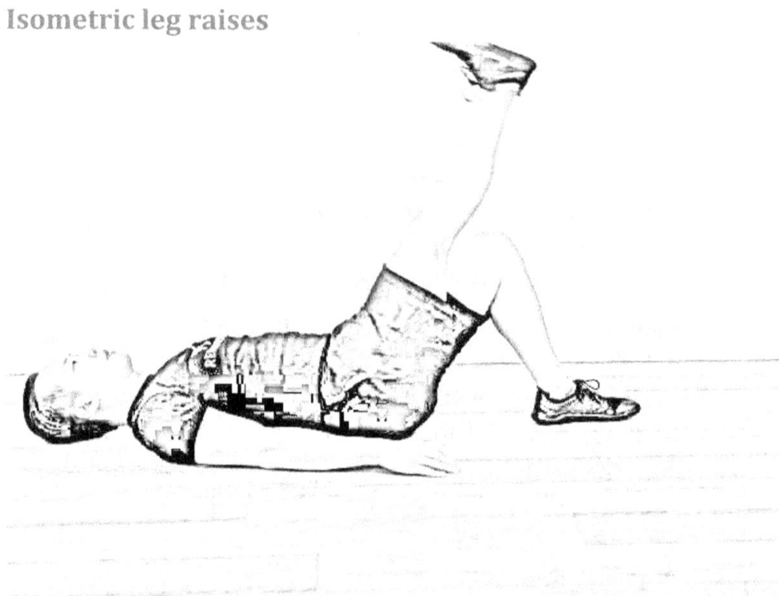

Isometric leg raises are an effective way to engage the lower body and core muscles without requiring complex movements. They focus on holding the legs in a fixed position, which creates a sustained contraction in the abdominal muscles and helps improve overall stability. When performed regularly, isometric leg raises can contribute to improved cardiovascular health, making them a beneficial exercise for individuals with high blood pressure.

Steps to Perform It:

1. **Lie down:** Begin by lying flat on your back on a mat or comfortable surface. Keep your legs straight and your arms by your sides for stability.
2. **Engage your core:** Tighten your abdominal muscles, ensuring your lower back stays flat on the ground.
3. **Lift your legs:** Slowly lift both legs together off the ground, keeping them straight, until they form about a 45-degree angle with your body.
4. **Hold the position:** Maintain this position for 15-30 seconds, keeping your core engaged and legs steady.
5. **Lower your legs:** After holding for the desired duration, slowly lower your legs back to the ground.
6. **Rest and repeat:** Rest for 30-60 seconds between repetitions, and then repeat the movement.

Frequency:

To manage high blood pressure, aim to perform isometric leg raises **2-3 times per week**. You can hold the position for 15 seconds, and increase gradually the duration as you build strength and endurance.

Benefits:

- **Improves core strength:** Isometric leg raises target the abdominal muscles, improving overall core stability and strength.
- **Supports blood pressure control:** Regular practice of this exercise can help in lowering resting blood pressure by engaging large muscle groups and improving circulation.

- **Strengthens lower body:** This exercise also engages the hip flexors and leg muscles, enhancing lower body strength and endurance.

Equipment Needed:

- No special equipment is required, but using a comfortable exercise mat can provide support.

Space Required:

- A small space is sufficient, roughly the size of your body lying flat on the ground.

Assistance Required:

- No assistance is typically needed, but beginners may benefit from supervision or feedback on proper form, especially when engaging the core muscles.

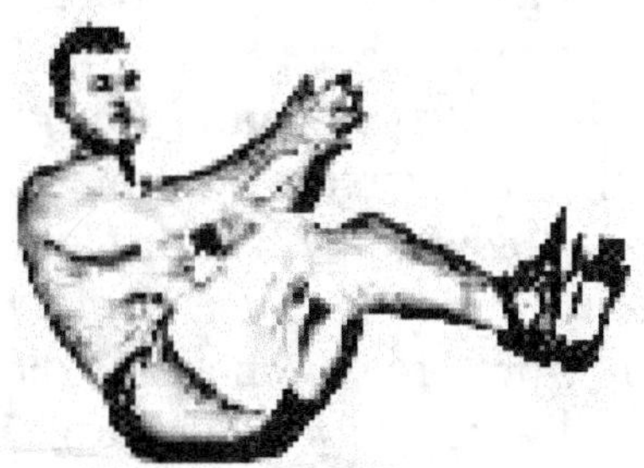

Isometric Russian Twists are a powerful way to strengthen your core muscles while supporting heart health through low-impact, controlled movements. The isometric hold during the twist helps maintain tension in the core, making this an effective exercise for both muscle toning and blood pressure management.

Steps to Perform It:

1. **Sit on the floor:** Begin by sitting on the floor with your knees bent and feet flat on the ground, hip-width apart.
2. **Lean back slightly:** Tilt your torso backward at a 45-degree angle, keeping your back straight to engage your core muscles.
3. **Lift your feet off the ground (optional):** For a more challenging version, lift your feet a few inches off the floor, balancing on your glutes.
4. **Clasp your hands together:** Bring your hands together in front of your chest or hold a light object (like a small weight) for added resistance.
5. **Twist slowly:** Rotate your torso to one side, keeping your arms extended. Hold this position for 15-30 seconds.
6. **Return to the center:** Slowly bring your torso back to the center and twist to the opposite side, holding again for 15-30 seconds.
7. **Complete the exercise:** Repeat for the desired number of sets, alternating sides.

Frequency:

To use isometric Russian twists for managing high blood pressure, aim to perform this exercise **2-3 times per week**. Beginners can start by holding each twist for 15 seconds per side and gradually build up to 30 seconds or more as their core strength improves.

Benefits:

*   **Improves core strength:** Isometric Russian twists engage the abdominal and oblique muscles,

strengthening the core and enhancing overall stability.
- **Supports cardiovascular health:** Like other isometric exercises, Russian twists can help in lowering blood pressure over time by improving circulation and reducing stress on the heart.
- **Enhances posture and balance:** Regular practice of this exercise helps improve spinal alignment and balance, reducing the risk of injury.
- **Increases flexibility:** Twisting motions help enhance the flexibility of the spine and the range of motion in the torso.

Equipment Needed:

- No equipment is required, but for an added challenge, a small weight, medicine ball, or resistance band can be used.

Space Required:

- You only need a small amount of space, about 4-5 feet, to comfortably perform the movement.

Assistance Required:

- No assistance is needed for this exercise, but beginners may benefit from a timer to keep track of hold durations or a mirror to ensure proper form.

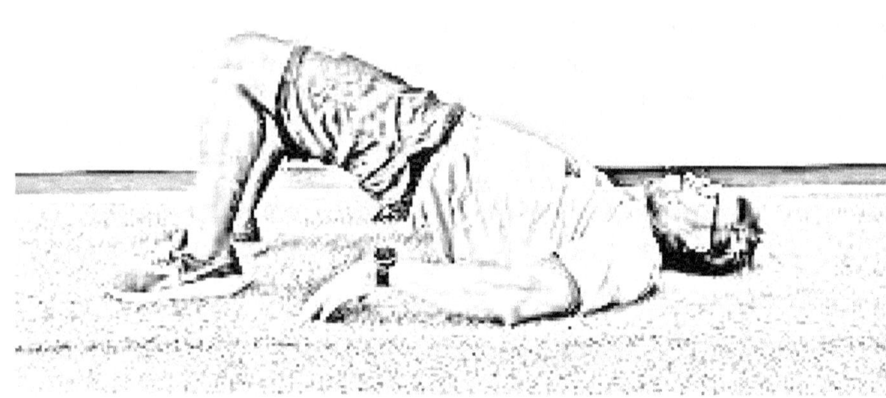

Isometric hip thrusts are an excellent exercise for targeting the glutes, hamstrings, and core, and they can be beneficial for people managing high blood pressure. This static exercise strengthens the lower body muscles while maintaining a steady heart rate, which is ideal for controlling blood pressure.

Steps to Perform It:

1. **Set up your position:**
   - Lie on your back with your knees bent and feet flat on the ground, about hip-width apart. Place your arms flat on the ground at your sides for balance.
2. **Lift your hips:**
   - Push through your heels and lift your hips toward the ceiling. A straight line should be formed by your body from your shoulders to your knees.
3. **Engage your core and glutes:**
   - Tighten your glutes and core muscles as you hold the position, keeping your hips elevated.
4. **Hold the position:**
   - Maintain the raised hip position for 15-30 seconds, or longer if you're able to.
5. **Lower back down:**
   - Slowly lower your hips to the starting position, then repeat the exercise.

Frequency:

To gain the benefits of isometric hip thrusts for lowering blood pressure, aim to do this exercise **2-3 times per week**. You can start with holding each thrust for 15 seconds, gradually building up to 30 seconds or more as your muscles strengthen.

Benefits:

- **Reduces blood pressure:** Holding the isometric contraction can help promote better blood circulation, which can lower resting blood pressure over time.

- **Strengthens lower body:** This exercise effectively targets the glutes, hamstrings, and core, which improves lower body strength.
- **Improves posture and stability:** Engaging the core during hip thrusts helps improve posture and enhances stability.
- **Boosts muscular endurance:** Holding the hip thrust position builds endurance in the glutes and hamstrings.

Equipment Needed:

- No equipment is required for this exercise, though an exercise mat is recommended for comfort.

Space Required:

- You only need a small area, about the size of your body lying down, to perform isometric hip thrusts.

Assistance Required:

- No assistance is required for this exercise. However, beginners might benefit from a mirror to ensure proper form.

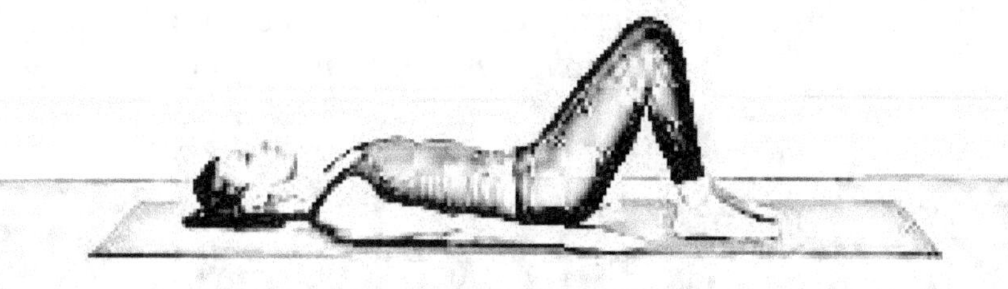

Isometric pelvic tilts are a simple but effective exercise that strengthens the lower back, abdominals, and pelvic muscles. These exercises also help reduce tension in the lower back and enhance posture, making them a beneficial addition to any routine aimed at lowering blood pressure.

Steps to Perform It:

1. **Lie down on your back:** Start by lying flat on your back on a mat or soft surface with your knees bent and feet flat on the ground.
2. **Engage your core:** Tighten your abdominal muscles as you press your lower back into the floor.
3. **Tilt your pelvis:** Slowly tilt your pelvis upward by tightening your glutes and lower abdominal muscles. This movement will cause your pelvis to slightly lift off the floor, flattening the small arch in your lower back.
4. **Hold the position:** Maintain this tilted position for 10-15 seconds, ensuring your back remains flat and your core stays engaged.
5. **Release:** After holding the position, slowly relax your muscles and return to the starting position.
6. **Repeat:** Perform the movement again for 5-10 repetitions, gradually increasing the hold time as you build strength.

Frequency:

To gain the blood pressure-lowering benefits of isometric pelvic tilts, aim to do the exercise **2-3 times per week**. Start with 5 repetitions per session, holding each pelvic tilt for about 10-15 seconds. As you get more comfortable, you can increase the duration to 20-30 seconds.

Benefits:

- **Strengthens the core and lower back:** Pelvic tilts engage the abdominal and lower back muscles, helping to strengthen and stabilize the core.

- **Improves posture:** Regular pelvic tilts can help enhance posture and reduce lower back discomfort by improving spinal alignment.
- **Lowers blood pressure:** Like other isometric exercises, isometric pelvic tilts can promote better circulation and reduce resting blood pressure.
- **Relieves tension:** This exercise helps alleviate tension in the hips, back, and pelvic region, making it useful for reducing stress.

Equipment Needed:

- None. You only need a soft surface like a yoga mat or towel to lie on.

Space Required:

- Minimal space is needed—just enough room to lie flat on your back with your legs bent.

Assistance Required:

- No assistance is typically needed to perform isometric pelvic tilts, but beginners may find it helpful to ask someone to guide them through the initial movements to ensure proper form.

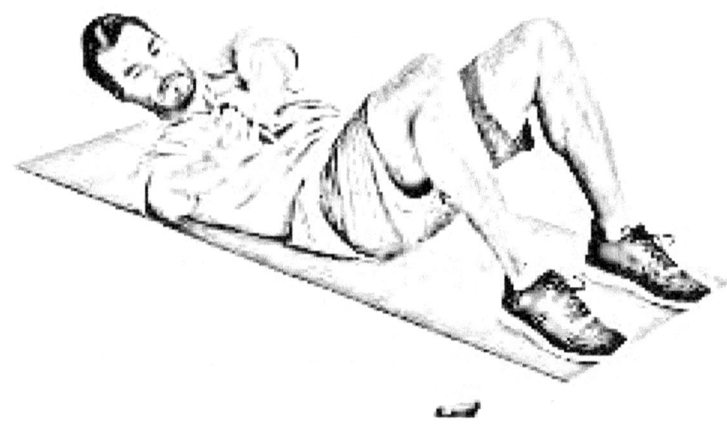

Isometric oblique twists target the oblique muscles, which are located on the sides of the abdomen. This exercise strengthens the core while remaining stationary during each twist. Unlike dynamic twisting exercises, the isometric version involves holding the twist at the end of the range of motion, helping to engage deep core muscles while reducing excessive movement that might raise blood pressure. It is a simple, yet highly effective, exercise for improving muscle endurance and supporting cardiovascular health.

Steps to Perform It:

1. **Start in a seated position:** Sit on the floor with your legs bent at the knees and feet flat on the ground.
2. **Lean back slightly:** Engage your core by leaning your torso back to about a 45-degree angle, ensuring your spine remains straight.
3. **Extend your arms:** Clasp your hands together in front of your chest or hold a light object (such as a small ball or weight).
4. **Perform the twist:** Slowly twist your torso to the right, keeping your arms extended and ensuring your hips stay still. Hold the position for 10-15 seconds.
5. **Return to the center:** After holding the position, return to the center and twist your torso to the left side, holding for the same amount of time.
6. **Repeat:** Alternate between both sides, keeping your core engaged throughout.

Frequency:

To manage high blood pressure effectively, perform isometric oblique twists **2-3 times per week** as part of your routine. Start by holding each twist for 10-15 seconds and gradually build up to longer holds as your strength improves.

Benefits:

- **Improves core strength:** Engages the oblique muscles and helps strengthen the entire core.
- **Enhances balance and stability:** By working on the core, this exercise promotes better balance and overall body stability.

- **Lowers blood pressure:** Regular isometric exercises like oblique twists can help lower resting blood pressure over time.
- **Supports good posture:** Strengthening the core helps maintain better posture and reduce strain on the back.

Equipment Needed:

- No equipment is required, though a light weight or medicine ball can be used to increase the intensity.

Space Required:

- A small space, around the size of a yoga mat, is sufficient for performing this exercise.

Assistance Required:

- Generally, no assistance is needed for this exercise, though beginners may find it helpful to have a timer or coach for monitoring their holds and form.

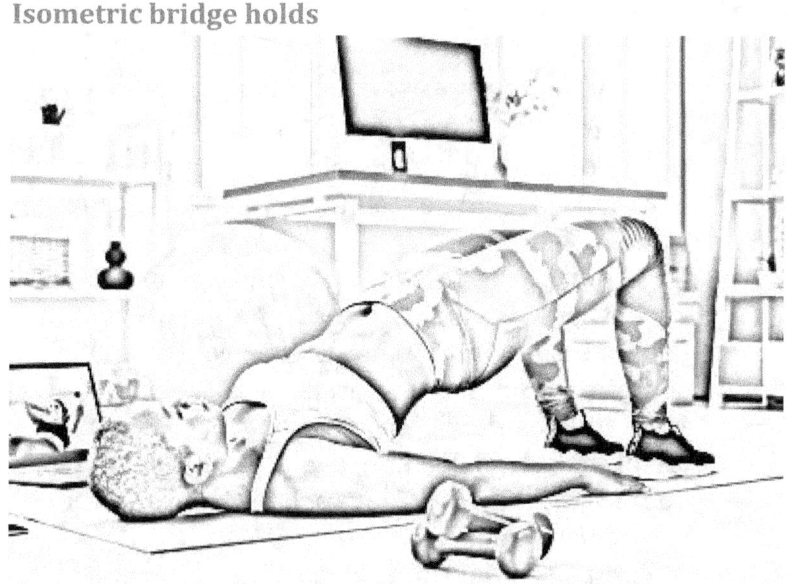

Isometric bridge holds are an effective way to engage multiple muscle groups, including the glutes, core, and lower back, while helping to reduce high blood pressure. By holding the bridge position without movement, you can improve muscle strength, endurance, and stability while promoting better circulation and reducing the overall workload on the cardiovascular system. This exercise is suitable for beginners and can be easily integrated into any workout routine

1. **Lie on your back:** Start by lying on your back on a mat or comfortable surface with your knees bent and feet flat on the floor, about hip-width apart. Your arms should be resting by your sides, palms facing down.
2. **Lift your hips:** Press through your feet and lift your hips toward the ceiling, creating a straight line from your knees to your shoulders. Engage your glutes and core muscles to support this movement.
3. **Hold the position:** Keep your body steady at the top of the bridge position, avoiding any arching of your lower back. Your knees, hips, and shoulders should be aligned.
4. **Breathe and maintain:** Focus on controlled breathing while holding this position for 15-30 seconds, depending on your strength level.
5. **Lower your hips:** Slowly lower your hips back down to the floor, keeping the movement controlled and smooth.
6. **Repeat:** Perform 2-4 sets, gradually increasing the hold time as you become stronger.

Frequency:

Incorporate isometric bridge holds into your routine **2-3 times per week**. Start with holding the bridge for 15 seconds and work your way up to 30 seconds or more. Ensure that you rest for about 30-60 seconds between sets.

Benefits:

- **Lowers blood pressure:** Regular performance of isometric bridge holds contributes to lowering resting blood pressure over time.

- **Strengthens core and lower body:** This exercise targets the glutes, hamstrings, and lower back, while also engaging the core.
- **Improves posture and stability:** Holding the bridge position helps develop muscle endurance and improves posture by strengthening the muscles supporting the spine.
- **Reduces muscle tension:** Isometric exercises like bridge holds promote blood flow and muscle relaxation, which can help relieve tension in the lower back.

Equipment Needed:

- A soft surface or mat for comfort while lying on the floor.

Space Required:

- A small space that allows you to lie down comfortably, around 6-7 feet of floor length.

Assistance Required:

- No assistance is required to perform isometric bridge holds, although beginners may benefit from using a timer or having someone assist with timing.

CHAPTER 6

Creating a Isometric Exercise Routine

Progressing Your Workouts Safely

Once you have established a solid foundation with beginner routines, it's essential to progress your workouts safely to continue reaping the benefits of isometric exercises. Listed below are the strategies which can also us do so

1. **Increase Hold Times**: Gradually increase the duration of each hold by 5-10 seconds every week. This progressive overload helps build strength without overwhelming your muscles.
2. **Add Variations**: Incorporate different variations of the same exercise to target different muscle groups. For example, if you've mastered wall sits, try adding arm raises or holding weights while in the position.
3. **Combine Isometric with Dynamic Movements**: For instance, you can perform a dynamic squat and hold at the bottom position for a few seconds before standing up. This combination challenges your muscles and enhances overall strength.
4. **Listen to Your Body**: Pay attention to how your body responds. If you experience discomfort or pain, reduce the intensity or duration of your holds. It's essential to avoid injury while progressing.
5. **Regularly Review Your Goals**: Set clear, achievable goals for your workouts, such as increasing the duration of your holds or the number of exercises you can perform. This will allow us to keep track.
6. **Consult a Professional**: If you're unsure how to progress safely, consider working with a fitness

professional who can tailor a program to your needs
and monitor your form.

Integrating isometric exercises into a broader fitness regimen can amplify their benefits, especially for individuals looking to manage high blood pressure. Here's how to effectively combine isometric workouts with other physical activities:

Cardiovascular Exercise

Incorporation: Combine isometric exercises with aerobic activities such as walking, jogging, cycling, or swimming. For instance, you could alternate between 20 minutes of brisk walking and 10 minutes of wall sits or push-up holds.

Benefits: Cardiovascular exercise helps improve heart health and blood circulation, while isometric workouts strengthen specific muscle groups. This combination can effectively lower blood pressure and enhance overall fitness.

Resistance Training

Incorporation: If you engage in traditional strength training, consider incorporating isometric holds into your routine. For example, during a bicep curl, hold the weight at the midpoint for several seconds before completing the movement.

Benefits: This approach can increase muscle engagement, leading to improved strength gains. Additionally, the isometric holds can help stabilize joints and reduce the risk of injury during dynamic movements.

Yoga and Pilates

Incorporation: Many yoga and Pilates poses involve isometric contractions. For instance, poses like the plank, warrior pose, or chair pose require you to hold your body in a fixed position, engaging various muscle groups isometrically.

Benefits: These practices improve flexibility, balance, and core strength while promoting relaxation and stress reduction, which are beneficial for managing blood pressure.

High-Intensity Interval Training (HIIT)

Incorporation: Integrate isometric exercises into a HIIT routine by alternating between high-intensity bursts of cardio (like sprinting or jumping jacks) and isometric holds (like planks or wall sits).

Benefits: HIIT workouts are efficient for burning calories and improving cardiovascular health. Adding isometric exercises enhances muscle endurance and strength while providing a different challenge to your muscles.

Functional Training

Incorporation: Functional training focuses on movements that mimic everyday activities. You can incorporate isometric exercises that enhance functional strength, like holding a lunge position or a squat.

Benefits: This training improves your ability to perform daily tasks and activities, contributing to overall health and independence, especially as you age.

Flexibility and Mobility Work

Incorporation: After your isometric workouts, incorporate stretching or mobility exercises to promote recovery and flexibility. Hold stretches for longer durations, incorporating isometric contractions by actively engaging the muscles while stretching.

Benefits: This practice can enhance muscle recovery, improve range of motion, and reduce muscle soreness.

Recovery Practices

Incorporation: After a rigorous workout, include isometric exercises in your recovery routine. For example, perform gentle isometric holds, like glute squeezes or abdominal contractions, while relaxing on a mat.

Benefits: Engaging in isometric exercises during recovery can facilitate blood flow to the muscles, aiding recovery without overexerting yourself.

CHAPTER 7

Monitoring Blood Pressure While Exercising

How to Measure Blood Pressure Accurately

Accurate blood pressure measurement is crucial for individuals managing hypertension, especially during and after exercise. Here's how to ensure accurate readings:

1. **Choosing the Right Equipment**:
   - **Automated Digital Monitors**: These are user-friendly and often recommended for home use. Ensure the device is validated for accuracy.
   - **Manual Sphygmomanometers**: If you prefer a manual method, it's essential to be trained in using this equipment correctly.
2. **Preparing for Measurement**:
   - **Rest Before Measurement**: Sit quietly for at least 5 minutes before taking a reading. This helps stabilize your blood pressure.
   - **Comfortable Position**: Sit with your back supported, feet flat on the floor, and arm at heart level.
   - **Avoid Stimulants**: Refrain from caffeine, nicotine, and vigorous exercise for at least 30 minutes prior to measurement.
3. **Technique for Measurement**:
   - **Cuff Placement**: Position the cuff on your upper arm, about an inch above the elbow crease. The cuff must not be tight but it can a snug a little.
   - **Take Multiple Readings**: For the most accurate results, take two or three readings, 1-2 minutes apart, and average them.

- o **Record the Measurements**: Keep a log of your readings, noting the date, time, and any relevant factors (e.g., before or after exercise).

4. **Measuring During Exercise**:
   - o **Timing**: If monitoring during exercise, take readings before starting, midway, and after the session. Use an automatic monitor designed for exercise settings, if possible.
   - o **Listen to Your Body**: If you experience dizziness, shortness of breath, or chest pain, stop exercising immediately and check your blood pressure.

Monitoring your progress in isometric exercises can help you understand the effectiveness of your routine and motivate you to continue. Here are some strategies:

1. **Keep a Workout Journal**:
    o **Document Exercises**: Write down the isometric exercises you perform, including the duration of each hold and the number of sets completed.
    o **Track Workouts**: Record any changes in routine, such as increased hold times or added variations.
2. **Monitor Blood Pressure Regularly**:
    o **Pre- and Post-Exercise Readings**: Measure your blood pressure before and after your workouts. This will help you assess how isometric exercise impacts your blood pressure levels.
    o **Record Trends**: Note any consistent changes over time, such as lower resting blood pressure readings.
3. **Set Specific Goals**:
    o **SMART Goals**: Establish Specific, Measurable, Achievable, Relevant, and Time-bound goals related to your isometric routine (e.g., "Increase wall sit hold from 20 seconds to 45 seconds within 4 weeks").
    o **Reassess Goals**: Regularly evaluate your progress and adjust your goals as needed.
4. **Use Technology**:
    o **Apps and Wearables**: Utilize fitness tracking apps or smartwatches that allow you to log workouts, monitor heart rate, and track blood pressure.

o **Regular Updates**: Sync your data regularly to observe trends and patterns in your progress.

As you incorporate isometric exercises into your routine, recognizing signs of improvement is vital for maintaining motivation and adjusting your program. Here are some indicators to look for:

1. **Lower Blood Pressure Readings**:
    o **Consistent Reductions**: If your blood pressure consistently decreases over weeks or months, this is a significant indicator that your exercise routine is effective.
    o **Improved Recovery Rates**: Notice if your blood pressure returns to baseline more quickly after exercise; this indicates improved cardiovascular health.
2. **Increased Strength and Endurance**:
    o **Longer Hold Times**: If you find that you can hold isometric positions for longer durations without fatigue, this is a clear sign of improved muscle strength and endurance.
    o **More Sets or Variations**: Being able to perform additional sets or incorporate more challenging variations of exercises also indicates progress.
3. **Enhanced Overall Fitness**:
    o **Increased Energy Levels**: Feeling more energetic and less fatigued during daily activities suggests that your fitness is improving.
    o **Better Performance in Other Activities**: If you notice improvements in your performance in other forms of exercise (like aerobic or resistance training), it indicates that isometric workouts are positively impacting your overall fitness.

4. **Physical Changes**:
    - o **Muscle Tone and Definition**: Look for visible changes in muscle tone or definition, particularly in the areas targeted by your isometric exercises.
    - o **Posture Improvement**: Enhanced core strength from isometric exercises may lead to better posture and alignment.
5. **Mental and Emotional Well-being**:
    - o **Reduced Stress Levels**: Many individuals report decreased stress and anxiety levels as they engage in regular physical activity. This can contribute to a positive feedback loop for exercise motivation.
    - o **Improved Mood and Confidence**: Enhanced mood, self-esteem, and confidence in your physical abilities can be powerful indicators of overall improvement.

CHAPTER 8

Lifestyle Modifications to Support Lower Blood Pressure

The Role of Diet in Hypertension Management

Diets serves an important role in managing blood pressure levels. Here are some dietary modifications that can help lower hypertension:

1. **Adopt the DASH Diet**:
   - **Dietary Approaches to Stop Hypertension (DASH)**: This eating plan emphasizes fruits, vegetables, whole grains, lean proteins, and low-fat dairy. The DASH diet is rich in potassium, calcium, and magnesium, which are beneficial for heart health.
   - **Limiting Sodium Intake**: Reducing sodium intake is crucial. Aim for less than 2,300 mg per day, or ideally, 1,500 mg, especially for those with high blood pressure. Focus on fresh foods and limit processed and packaged foods, which are often high in salt.
2. **Increase Fiber Intake**:
   - **Fruits and Vegetables**: Aim for at least five servings of fruits and vegetables each day. These foods are not only low in calories but also high in dietary fiber, which can help lower blood pressure.
   - **Whole Grains**: Incorporate whole grains like brown rice, oats, and quinoa, which are high in fiber and nutrients.
3. **Choose Healthy Fats**:

- o **Unsaturated Fats**: Replace saturated fats with healthy fats, such as those found in olive oil, avocados, nuts, and fatty fish (like salmon and mackerel), which contain omega-3 fatty acids.
  - o **Limit Trans Fats**: Avoid trans fats found in many processed foods, as they can raise cholesterol levels and increase the risk of heart disease.

4. **Moderate Alcohol Consumption**:
   - o **Alcohol and Blood Pressure**: While some studies suggest that moderate alcohol consumption may have heart benefits, excessive drinking can raise blood pressure.

5. **Reduce Added Sugars**:
   - o **Sugar and Blood Pressure**: High sugar consumption, particularly from sugary drinks and snacks, can contribute to obesity and increased blood pressure. Opt for natural sources of sweetness, like fruits, instead of added sugars.

6. **Stay Hydrated**:
   - o **Water Intake**: Proper hydration supports overall cardiovascular health. Aim to drink plenty of water throughout the day, and consider herbal teas or other non-caffeinated, non-sugary beverages.

Chronic stress is a significant contributor to elevated blood pressure. Implementing effective stress management techniques can support blood pressure control:

1. **Mindfulness and Meditation**:
   - **Practice Mindfulness**: Engaging in mindfulness techniques, such as meditation, can help reduce stress and promote relaxation. Always target at least 10-15 minutes of meditation daily.
   - **Breathing Exercises**: Simple deep-breathing exercises can lower heart rate and blood pressure. Practice inhaling deeply for four counts, holding for four, and exhaling for six counts.
2. **Regular Physical Activity**:
   - **Exercise as a Stress Reliever**: Regular physical activity can significantly reduce stress levels. Incorporate a mix of aerobic activities and isometric exercises into your routine for optimal benefits.
   - **Outdoor Activities**: Spending time in nature or engaging in outdoor activities can enhance mood and alleviate stress.
3. **Social Support**:
   - **Connect with Others**: Maintaining strong social connections can provide emotional support and reduce feelings of stress. Engage in regular social activities or communicate with friends and family.
   - **Seek Professional Help**: If stress becomes overwhelming, consider talking to a mental health professional for support and coping strategies.

4. **Time Management**:
    o   **Organizing Tasks**: Effective time management can reduce stress related to feeling overwhelmed. Learn by dividing larger tasks into small task.
    o   **Create Downtime**: Schedule regular breaks throughout your day to rest and recharge. Allocating time for hobbies and relaxation can help manage stress levels.
5. **Healthy Coping Mechanisms**:
    o   **Avoid Unhealthy Habits**: Avoid resorting to unhealthy coping mechanisms, such as smoking or excessive alcohol consumption, which can increase blood pressure. Instead, find healthier outlets, such as exercise, art, or journaling.

Quality sleep and adequate rest are essential components of overall health, particularly for managing blood pressure. Here's how to optimize sleep for cardiovascular well-being:

1. **Prioritize Sleep Hygiene**:
   - **Establish a Routine**: Go to bed and wake up at the same time each day to regulate your body's internal clock. If you have a consistent sleep schedule, it will enhance sleep quality.
   - **Create a Restful Environment**: Ensure your bedroom is conducive to sleep—cool, dark, and quiet. Always minimize distractions using blackout curtains, earplugs, or white noise machines.
2. **Limit Stimulants**:
   - **Caffeine and Nicotine**: Reduce or eliminate consumption of caffeine and nicotine, especially in the afternoon and evening, as they can interfere with your ability to fall asleep.
   - **Screen Time**: Limit exposure to screens (phones, computers, TVs) at least an hour before bed.
3. **Relaxation Techniques**:
   - **Wind Down**: Establish a calming pre-sleep routine. Activities such as reading, taking a warm bath, or practicing gentle stretching can signal to your body that it's time to relax.
   - **Mindfulness Before Bed**: Engage in relaxation techniques such as meditation, deep breathing, or progressive muscle

relaxation to ease tension and prepare for sleep.

4. **Address Sleep Disorders**:
   - **Sleep Apnea Awareness**: If you suspect you have a sleep disorder like sleep apnea, seek medical advice. Sleep apnea can contribute to hypertension and increase the risk of cardiovascular issues.
   - **Consult a Professional**: If you have persistent trouble sleeping, consider consulting a healthcare professional for evaluation and possible treatment options.
5. **Monitor Sleep Quality**:
   - **Use Sleep Trackers**: Consider using wearable devices or apps to monitor your sleep patterns. These tools can help you identify factors affecting your sleep quality and allow you to make necessary adjustments.

CHAPTER 9

Special Considerations for Specific Populations

Isometric Exercise for Seniors

As people age, maintaining physical health becomes increasingly vital, especially regarding blood pressure management. Isometric exercises can be particularly beneficial for seniors due to their low-impact nature and ease of incorporation into daily routines.

1. **Benefits of Isometric Exercise for Seniors**:
   o **Muscle Strength and Endurance**: Isometric exercises help maintain and build muscle strength, which is essential for daily activities and overall functional independence.
   o **Joint Health**: These exercises place less strain on the joints compared to dynamic movements, making them suitable for seniors who may experience joint pain or arthritis.
   o **Improved Blood Pressure Control**: Regular isometric exercises have been shown to positively impact blood pressure, making them a valuable tool for managing hypertension in older adults.
2. **Recommended Isometric Exercises**:
   o **Wall Sits**: Standing against a wall and sliding down until the knees are at a 90-degree angle strengthens the quadriceps and glutes.
3. **Safety Considerations**:
   o **Consult with Healthcare Providers**: Seniors should always consult with their

healthcare provider before starting any new exercise routine, especially if they have pre-existing conditions.

- o **Focus on Proper Form**: Emphasizing correct posture and form can help prevent injury. Utilizing mirrors or having a partner assist can be beneficial.

4. **Incorporating Isometric Exercises into Daily Routine**:
   - o **Routine Integration**: Encourage seniors to incorporate isometric exercises into their daily activities, such as performing wall sits while watching television or doing hand presses during meals.
   - o **Social Engagement**: Group exercise classes focused on isometric movements can provide both physical and social benefits, fostering community and motivation.

For individuals with heart conditions, incorporating exercise into their lifestyle is crucial for managing health. Isometric exercises can offer a safe and effective way to improve cardiovascular health without excessive strain.

1. **Understanding Heart Conditions and Exercise**:
   - **Consultation is Key**: Individuals with heart conditions should always consult their healthcare provider or a cardiologist before beginning any exercise program to ensure safety and suitability.
   - **Monitoring Heart Rate**: Keeping track of heart rate during exercise can help gauge intensity and ensure that it remains within a safe range.
2. **Benefits of Isometric Exercises for Heart Patients**:
   - **Low Impact**: Isometric exercises minimize the risk of sudden spikes in heart rate, making them safer for individuals with heart conditions.
   - **Strengthening the Heart**: Engaging in regular isometric exercises can help improve overall muscle strength, which indirectly supports heart health by reducing the workload on the heart.
3. **Recommended Isometric Exercises**:
   - **Seated Arm Presses**: While seated, individuals can press their palms together in front of their chest or against a sturdy surface to engage upper body muscles.
   - **Leg Presses Against a Wall**: Sitting against a wall, individuals can push their heels into

the ground, creating tension in the leg muscles without straining the heart.
   o **Isometric Core Exercises**: Gentle isometric core exercises, such as holding a seated position with a straight back, can help improve stability without undue strain.
4. **Progression and Monitoring**:
   o **Start Slowly**: Begin with short sessions (5-10 minutes) and gradually increase duration and intensity as tolerated, ensuring regular check-ins with a healthcare provider.
   o **Recognize Warning Signs**: Be aware of warning signs, such as dizziness, chest pain, or shortness of breath, and stop exercising immediately if any arise.

Individuals with limited mobility may face unique challenges when incorporating exercise into their routines, but isometric exercises can be adapted to suit their needs.

1. **Benefits of Isometric Exercises for Limited Mobility**:
   o **Accessibility**: Isometric exercises can be performed seated or lying down, making them accessible for those with limited mobility.
   o **Strength Building**: These exercises help maintain or build muscle strength without requiring extensive movement, which can be particularly beneficial for those with disabilities or recovering from injury.
2. **Recommended Modifications**:
   o **Seated Exercises**: Many isometric exercises can be performed while seated in a sturdy chair, such as seated arm presses, leg extensions, or seated torso twists.
   o **Lying Down Exercises**: Individuals can perform isometric contractions while lying down, such as pressing the arms against the floor or holding a plank position with the knees on the ground.
   o **Adaptive Equipment**: Use of resistance bands or therapy balls can provide additional support and help engage muscles without requiring full mobility.
3. **Creating a Safe Environment**:
   o **Safety First**: Ensure that the exercise space is safe and accessible, free of clutter, and equipped with necessary aids like grab bars or sturdy furniture for support.

- o **Use of Chairs and Support Devices**: Incorporating supportive devices can assist individuals in maintaining balance and stability during exercises.
4. **Incorporating Caregivers or Support**:
   - o **Partner Workouts**: Encourage family members or caregivers to join in the exercise routine. This can provide motivation and ensure safety during the workouts.
   - o **Professional Guidance**: Collaborating with physical therapists or occupational therapists can help design tailored exercise programs that cater to individual needs and limitations.

CHAPTER 10

Common Misconceptions About Isometric Exercise

Isometric exercise, while effective for many individuals, is often surrounded by myths and misconceptions. Understanding the truth behind these can help individuals make informed decisions about their fitness routines.

1. **Myth: Isometric Exercise Is Ineffective for Building Muscle**
   - **Reality**: While isometric exercises do not produce the same muscle growth as dynamic exercises, they are effective for increasing muscle endurance and strength. Research indicates that regular isometric training can lead to improvements in muscle performance and hypertrophy when incorporated into a balanced workout regimen.
2. **Myth: Isometric Exercise Is Only for Athletes**
   - **Reality**: Isometric exercises are accessible to everyone, regardless of fitness level. They can be easily modified for beginners or individuals with limited mobility, making them suitable for seniors or those recovering from injury.
3. **Myth: Isometric Exercises Are Dangerous for Individuals with High Blood Pressure**
   - **Reality**: While it's true that certain exercises can increase blood pressure temporarily, isometric exercises, when performed correctly and under medical guidance, can be safe and beneficial for individuals with

hypertension. It's essential to focus on proper breathing and technique.

4. **Myth: You Need Specialized Equipment for Isometric Exercise**
    - **Reality**: Many isometric exercises can be performed using just body weight or simple household items. For example, wall sits or static lunges can be done without any equipment, making isometric exercises highly accessible.

A common question arises about the effectiveness of isometric exercise as an alternative to hypertension medication.

1. **Understanding Blood Pressure Management**:
   - **Holistic Approach**: Managing high blood pressure typically requires a comprehensive approach, including lifestyle modifications (diet, exercise, stress management), regular monitoring, and sometimes medication. Isometric exercise can be a valuable component of this strategy, but it is not a standalone solution.
2. **Research Findings**:
   - **Supplementary Role**: Studies have shown that isometric exercise can lead to reductions in blood pressure comparable to those achieved with some antihypertensive medications. However, this does not mean that it can replace medication for everyone. The effectiveness varies by individual and health status.
3. **Consulting Healthcare Providers**:
   - **Personalized Plans**: It is crucial for individuals to work closely with their healthcare providers to develop a personalized plan. Some individuals may find that incorporating isometric exercises alongside their prescribed medications can enhance their blood pressure management.
4. **Potential Risks of Discontinuing Medication**:
   - **Risk Awareness**: Stopping medication without consulting a doctor can lead to

dangerous spikes in blood pressure. Individuals should always seek medical advice before making changes to their treatment plans.

The timeline for seeing results from isometric exercise can vary widely depending on individual circumstances, including frequency of workouts, starting fitness level, and overall health.

1. **Initial Benefits**:
    - **Short-Term Effects**: Many individuals report feeling stronger and more stable within a few weeks of beginning an isometric exercise routine. Improvements in muscle endurance and joint stability can often be felt relatively quickly.
2. **Blood Pressure Changes**:
    - **Longer Timeline**: While some studies indicate that regular isometric training can lead to noticeable reductions in blood pressure within 4 to 8 weeks, individual responses can vary. Factors such as diet, stress levels, and adherence to the exercise program also play significant roles.
3. **Consistency Is Key**:
    - **Regular Practice**: For optimal results, consistency is vital. Engaging in isometric exercises at least 2-3 times a week can help ensure sustained improvements in blood pressure and overall fitness.
4. **Monitoring Progress**:
    - **Tracking Changes**: Individuals should monitor their blood pressure regularly to track changes and assess the effectiveness of their exercise routine. Keeping a journal of workouts and results can also help identify patterns and areas for improvement.
5. **Patience and Realistic Expectations**:

- o **Mindset Matters**: It's essential to have realistic expectations when starting any exercise program. While improvements may take time, committing to a consistent routine can yield significant long-term benefits for blood pressure and overall health

CHAPTER 11

Conclusion

Isometric exercise emerges as a powerful tool in the quest to manage high blood pressure, offering a safe, effective, and accessible form of physical activity that can complement traditional treatment methods. By focusing on muscle contractions without movement, isometric exercises not only enhance muscle strength and endurance but also contribute to cardiovascular health by promoting reductions in blood pressure levels.

Throughout this book, we have explored the myriad benefits of incorporating isometric exercises into daily routines, emphasizing their adaptability for various populations, including seniors, individuals with heart conditions, and those with limited mobility. The flexibility of isometric training makes it an ideal choice for anyone seeking to improve their health without the risks associated with more vigorous activities.

Furthermore, it is essential to recognize that while isometric exercise can significantly aid in blood pressure management, it should be part of a holistic approach that includes a balanced diet, stress management, and regular monitoring of one's health. Consulting healthcare providers ensures that individuals can tailor their exercise routines to their specific needs, making informed choices that prioritize safety and efficacy.

In conclusion, embracing isometric exercise as a valuable addition to a lifestyle aimed at lowering blood pressure empowers individuals to take control of their health. By fostering consistency and commitment, individuals can experience improved strength, endurance, and overall well-being. With the right guidance and a positive mindset, isometric exercise can pave the way toward a healthier, more vibrant life, ultimately contributing to the successful management of hypertension.